Love in the
Next 10 Seconds

Love in the Next 10 Seconds

Changing the Box of Relationship
Into Living Without Limits

Nirmada Kaufman

&

John Andros

RADICAL
DEMAND

ISBN: 978-0-9963964-7-9
eBook: 978-0-9963964-1-7

Printed and bound in San Francisco by Radical Demand, Inc.

We dedicate this book to Gary Douglas, Dr. Dain Heer, and all the seekers in the world who know that something else is possible and are choosing it.

ACKNOWLEDGMENTS

~

First and foremost, we would like to express our gratitude and thanks to you, Gary Douglas, the founder of Access Consciousness®, for your enormous contributions that have expanded our lives, our relationship, our awareness, and for the creation of new possibilities on Earth.

Thank you for creating the tools and processes that are presented in this book, and for contributing to creating a World that we desire to live in. You have always inspired us to be ourselves and to create something greater, and for this we will always be grateful.

Thank you with gratitude to Dr. Dain Heer, co-creator of Access Consciousness. Your brilliant facilitation, the creation of the "Symphony of Possibilities" and your kindness and vulnerability have changed our lives and contributed greatly to the creation of this book.

We would also like to thank and acknowledge Access Consciousness for its phenomenal tools and processes that are now changing lives in over 175 countries. Its tools are presented throughout these pages and have allowed us to create this book as our gift to you, the reader.

We are so grateful to you, Earth, for allowing us to consciously grow and thrive on beautiful you.

We would like to thank our families for always supporting us.

We are infinitely grateful to you, Sage Lee, for your friendship, wisdom and brilliant business coaching, which have enriched our lives and contributed greatly to the creation of this book.

Thank you with gratitude to Sasha Allenby and Lois Rose. We appreciate your immense dedication and contributions to the creation of this book.

Acknowledgments

And thank you with gratitude to the entire Access Consciousness Worldwide Team for being brilliant creators. Thank you as well to Sharee Alchin Photography and everyone else that has contributed, directly or indirectly, to this book.

We also desire to give special thanks to all the amazing people who are willing to create a different possibility for living harmoniously here on Earth.

CONTENTS

~

PART TWO
Practicing the Tools For a New Kind of Relationship

PART THREE
Creating The Future You Really Desire

FOREWORD

~

In all of us there seems to be the search for someone or something that validates, inspires and invigorates our lives and shows us that we have value to the world.

Nirmada and John are two people who have been on this search and have found the way that works to make living more joyful with each other than without.

I think this book may awaken the awareness for some, that there can be, and will be, a different world if we choose it. Making a relationship that works for you is a great gift and this is what Nirmada and John wish to invite all of you to become aware of and be able to choose.

May this voice in the darkness be the gift you deserve and light you are looking for.

Gary Douglas
Founder of Access Consciousness

INTRODUCTION

~

Journey into a
New Paradigm of Relationship

WE IMAGINE THAT you picked up this book because you are asking for a change.

The thing that you bought into up until now, called 'relationship,' may no longer be serving you. Maybe you even feel that it never really served you in the first place.

Perhaps you have been seeking something radically different. Or perhaps, on some level, you know that it's possible to have something different, but you haven't known how to create it for yourself. Have you found that you keep experiencing more of the same, however hard you have tried to change? Perhaps the characters and names have changed, but, up until now, the game itself has remained the same.

Have you noticed, from the moment we arrive in this World, how we are programmed into making it significant whether someone loves us or not? How much of this programming comes from the movies we see and the love songs we hear? You may have found yourself shaping these 'programs' into the things that we call 'love and relationship'.

If you have played this game, and are now reading this book, chances are it probably doesn't work for you anymore. How much of this old paradigm of relationship has kept you locked into seeking the approval from another in order to be validated? What if you could just be yourself regardless of who is in your life or not?

Many people find that in this old scenario they are not able to be themselves. An expression we use to describe this situation is "cutting off parts and pieces of ourselves" in order to stay in a relationship. Have you found yourself cutting off parts and pieces of you in order to stay with someone, rather than just being yourself?

Much of what we have been taught in the old paradigm of relationship has revolved around 'wrongness'. Have you ever found that you've learned to make your partner wrong, gathering evidence and sharing with others why you thought they were wrong, so that you could be right?

Many relationships in the old paradigm focus on whether the other person was 'right or wrong' or 'good or bad'. In this scenario, if you believed your partner was right or good, did you reward them? If you believed they were wrong or bad, did you push them away? It's most likely that you have also been on the receiving end of this scenario.

So, what if you no longer had to make your partner wrong? What if you no longer made yourself wrong either? Getting out of the old paradigm of 'right' or 'wrong' in relationship is one of the evolutionary changes being offered to you here in this book.

An Evolutionary New Paradigm

We are presenting you with a radically new approach for creating your life and relationship. You may have noticed that we started asking you questions right from the beginning. Learning to ask questions empowers you to change old patterns that are no longer working for you. Asking questions also creates an evolutionary new paradigm, both in your life, and in your relationship. With this in mind, we would like to ask: "If you could have anything from this book, what would it be?"

First and foremost, this is not a book of answers about how to 'do' relationship. This book and our approach are profoundly different from the old paradigm of relationship counseling where someone tells you what you should do in order to be happy. Instead, it is about supporting you in your own awareness of what is going to work for you, and empowering you to create this for yourself. Ultimately, nobody else's answer is greater than your own awareness.

We have found that the tools presented in this book have worked for many people around the world, as they are based on asking questions and not on giving answers. All the way through this book we are going to be asking you questions and sharing practical tools that will empower you to create a life and relationship that work for you.

What if You Could Be Empowered to Know that *You* Know?

We are going to show you how to ask questions in a way that allows you to get out of conclusions and into trusting your own awareness. Conclusions are the fixed points of view that prevent us from creating or experiencing anything beyond our current reality.

Any of us who have had a relationship in the old paradigm are likely to have had some kind of "conclusionary reality" programmed into us. This is where we have taken on the opinions, beliefs and judgments of others about relationship and adopted them as our own.

You will learn how to change this by asking questions, such as "Is this really true for me?" or "Is this really my point of view?" or "Did I just buy it as true?" The tools in this book will enable you to become more aware of what's not working for you and to learn how to choose what does work for you.

In the new paradigm, there is no 'right' or 'wrong' way to do relationship. How freeing does this feel to you, knowing that you would no longer have to try to figure it out or to get it right?

At no point in this book are any of the tools and concepts about making you, your partner or your relationship wrong. Instead, you will be empowered and encouraged to ask questions such as "What else is possible?" and learn to create your new paradigm of relationship.

You will be guided to ask: "What can I change here?", when something isn't working. You will learn a way of asking questions that allows you to change the things that aren't working for you and create more harmony in the process.

Making Choices in 10-Second Increments

What if you could, as the title of this book suggests, create your life and relationship 10 seconds at a time? What if you could make a choice, and if it doesn't work out, then instead of going into judgment or wrongness, you could simply make a new choice in the next 10 seconds?

We know that asking questions isn't new. However, the way we are going to show you how to ask questions is a radically different approach to what you may have learned before. This approach will allow you to get out of functioning from your fixed points of view about how your life or relationship 'should' be, and into learning how to create your new paradigm of living without limits.

By now, you may have heard countless times that you can create your own reality. However, how many people do you know that are actually doing this? *Love in the Next 10 Seconds* will guide you on being the creator of your own reality; we will show you how to expand every area in your life and relationship.

Before you dive into this journey with us, we are going to share our own relationship story with you, and we'll also share what has occurred for us as we have applied the tools contained in this book. We'll take you right to the beginning, where we first met, so you can see our own evolution.

Nirmada and John's Story

NIRMADA: "What contribution can I be to ease the pain between men and women on this planet?"

It was the question that I asked myself on the night that everything in my life turned around.

You may have encountered a night similar to the one that I had, in your own life. A night where everything that you have known or believed to be true for you crumbles before your eyes and you are left stripped bare and you have nothing left to cling to. Some people call these moments 'the dark night of the soul', but for me it would be more accurate to describe it as a moment that was to shape my future and the way I lived from that moment onwards.

The catalyst for the turning point occurred during a body class I was attending. The teacher spoke about very different possibilities that are available for men and women to relate to one another — possibilities that confront almost every aspect of our current concept of relationship.

As I was listening intently to the teacher, I knew emphatically that what he was saying was true for me. And then, a woman in the class made fun of what had been said and other people laughed, agreeing with her. The teacher considered this to be unacceptable and swore that he would never speak about the subject again. The concepts he had shared were so valuable to mankind — it was inconceivable to me that this information would no longer be available.

When I got back to my room, I was called to face myself in a way that I'd never done before: to examine the far reaches of the paradigm that I had called 'relationship' in this lifetime, and turn it upside down.

That night, I went into meltdown.

It wasn't the kind of meltdown you would associate with hopelessness or despair. It was more of a deep knowing that everything needed to dissolve before it could be created again. A new choice was born. In fact, it was more like a demand. From that moment forward, I was going to do things in a different way — for myself, and for all the men and women on this planet who are disharmonious and distraught in the way they relate to each other.

The new choice emerging was to contribute ways of changing to all the men and women who have been trying to conform to a predetermined and outdated definition of what relationship is supposed to be like, even though it no longer serves them.

And, it was for all the men and women who were, like me, asking to not go around in those same tired old patterns anymore. And, it was for all those who desire freedom, growth, and harmony in their relationships and know it is possible and just don't know how to actually create it.

What I have seen in the vast majority of people I have encountered is that, however sophisticated or evolved they are in their lives as a whole, that same level of sophistication and harmony isn't reflected in their connection in relationship. And I knew that it was time for this to change!

Three weeks after I stood there and declared to the universe that I was demanding something different in relationship, John appeared in my life.

JOHN: The first thing Nirmada ever said to me was: "Take off your clothes!"

Well, to be more precise, it wasn't directed personally at me, but to everyone in the volcanic hot springs where we met.

As I approached the springs I heard her say: "Anyone who comes in here has to be naked." She was taking all the women's bikini tops off, and by the time I got there, she was insisting that the men get naked too. The thing to understand about Nirmada is that there was a total freedom and innocence in the way she beckoned people into the springs that day.

And it enabled everyone to be at ease with themselves as a result. All the barriers that people usually associate with getting naked in front of a bunch of strangers seemed to dissolve. By her very playful nature she invited others to be uninhibited and free.

When we began to talk, the first thing I noticed was how easy the connection was. There were no barriers, no judgments, no expectations, no games, and no measuring each other up. Just a complete allowance for the other person to show up exactly as they were.

Up until I met Nirmada, I would say that I'd been 'settling'. I was still in a relationship at that point, but it was one that was gradually falling apart. It kind of worked, on some level, but there was a quiet suppression of what was true for me, as we went through the motions of what we had built together in the past. We were married, with two teenage children in the picture. We had made a half-hearted commitment to stay together, with the agreement that we could start seeing other people. Despite this agreement, I hadn't been with anyone else.

So this is how I arrived in Costa Rica for the seven-day *Celebration of Life and Living* event where I met Nirmada. And even though my work at the time reflected the same pattern of settling that I'd fallen into with my previous relationship (I was working in the mines in Australia), and there was little money in the bank, there had been a really strong sense of being 'called' to this class. I'd traveled halfway around the world with the deep knowing that I just had to be there. In hindsight, I now know why.

NIRMADA: One of the first things I noticed about the way that John and I communicated was the level of vulnerability we had with each other. We just showed up and allowed each other to be.

As there was such ease between us, we were able to contribute to each other and receive from each other in a way that I had never experienced before. The class we were attending contributed to the deepening of our shared awareness of a new possibility in relationship.

Part of the process in the class was to support changes in the physical body, and one of the practices was "body trades", where participants facilitated changes for one another. This was a silent, hands-on practice, and it was natural for me to ask John if he wanted to trade.

The experience was incredible. We traded all day, gifting and receiving. Each of our bodies was totally aware of the other, and something tremendously powerful occurred for both of us in those moments.

It soon became apparent that what was taking place between us was also contributing to many others in the class. People commented to us that the connection between us was enabling a deeper connection between other attendees. It was as though our combined presence changed the whole room.

It became evident, in those very early moments of being together, that we were already influencing those around us with the communion we were experiencing with each other.

When I saw John after class, two things were glaringly obvious to me. The first was that there was something really different going on with us. The second was that I knew I was the one who had to make a move here. So, discarding any preconceived gender roles, I invited him to my room.

JOHN: I knew, the moment I accepted the invitation to go to Nirmada's room, that everything was going to unravel.

There was such a contrast between where Nirmada was and where I was then. She had been divorced for ten years and single, and my external world was still very much tied up in a marriage that wasn't working. My children, my job, and my life were on the other side of the world.

Even though there was that agreement with my previous partner for both of us to have an open relationship (as long as we used condoms), this wasn't something I was going to enter into lightly.

I had always been pretty highly turned on. But something inside me had always ensured that I thought about consequences before I took action. I'd learned to control the basic male tendency to 'fool around first' and then deal with the consequences later.

In more recent years, I'd learned four questions (we'll share more about these with you later) that I asked myself before choosing to have sex with a person. They are: "Will it be fun?" and "Will it be easy?" and "Will I learn something?" and "Will they be grateful?" Up until the point I met Nirmada, I had asked myself these questions in regard to more than 100 different women and had never gotten a 'yes' to all four of them.

My impression is that the majority of men in the current paradigm of sex and relationship may not ask these questions, and even if they did ask these questions and did not get a 'yes' to all four, they would probably override this fact, and still go ahead, dealing with the consequences and subsequent fallout later.

It's never seemed "light" for me to override my awareness when I don't get a 'yes' to all four questions (and we'll explore how you know something is "light" for you as we go through this book). However, when I asked myself these four questions about Nirmada, I got a straight 'yes' for all four.

Despite this, I didn't instantly want to have sex with her. I was still uncertain. One of the things I appreciated about Nirmada at that time was that she gave me so much space. There was such an honoring of where I was at, and this in turn created a deep trust. It was the turning point of our connection.

NIRMADA: I totally honored John's choice not to have sex at that point. I was very aware of where he was at and what he required. Just as I'd had my moment three weeks prior where everything had unraveled in my awareness, just as much was unraveling for John, particularly in his external world.

He was in a relationship that was just about over. He hadn't taken legal steps to separate, but it was obvious from the outside that it was at that stage. There was none of the old paradigm of getting my needs met in order to be validated (which is the driver for so many people in a situation such as the one we were experiencing).

We had a beautiful night of lying there naked in each other's presence and having gratitude for each other. He told me the next morning: "You truly gained my trust because you had so much allowance for where I was at."

What occurred after that night was also a reflection of the choice we had given each other in that first, naked encounter in my room. At every stage thereafter, we also gave each other choice, and we still do, to this day.

We didn't assume, for example, that because we had spent the night together naked, that we would be trade partners again the next day in class. We made it about choice. Just as on that first night, it was about choice when I asked him, "Would you like to spend the night here or would you like to go back to your room?" Again, there were no assumptions, as it all came down to choice.

In fact, this kind of choosing—moment by moment or 10 seconds at a time, as the title of this book suggests— is at the heart of what enables our connection to work. It is at the core of what we will be sharing with you in this book, and one of the key tools that will enable you to turn your current relationship paradigm into new possibilities.

Right from the start, we ensured that every single choice that each of us made individually was one that was made from awareness. Later we will share with you how this kind of choosing differs from a fixed commitment in relationship, and how you can apply it to your own relationship, to experience more ease, joy and harmony.

JOHN: The next night we chose to stay together again and this time we did make love. There was such a flow of energy between us. Our bodies loved being together. It was instantly apparent that we were experiencing an "energetic match". Our bodies were so receptive to one another.

Everything sexual I desired to have, I received that night, and I didn't even have to ask for it! And it was the same for Nirmada. We realized later how much our bodies had been deprived of such a high level of contribution. It was a communion on every level.

During that night, every cell in my body felt like it was vitally alive. My senses were heightened to an extraordinary level. After having sex, I lay there listening to the sounds of the Costa Rican jungle. One thing I remember vividly was the screeching of a group of monkeys that surrounded our cabin. It made the whole experience even more primal as they howled around us.

We continued to choose to do body trades in class. It was as though our bodies were one note. With my eyes closed, I'd move my arm up to a certain point, and find that Nirmada's hand was exactly above that place waiting for my hand. I instinctively knew where her hands were, even when they weren't touching my body.

People started to notice how what we were creating together was having a profound effect on the whole class. What was occurring in that class was a microcosm for the work we would later be drawn to do with others, and a reflection of our greater calling together. Many people told us that our way of connecting in class allowed them also to have a greater sense of communion. (This is part of what we are going to share with you in this book.)

From then on, we knew that we had walked through a door together and there was no going back. We lived on opposite sides of the world. To us, although there were a lot of logistics to work through on one level, it was an easier choice to make than you might imagine.

What we were actually doing—something that we are going to be sharing how to do as this book progresses—was asking questions and perceiving what was energetically light for us, and choosing that. We were, and still are, simply following the energy and making choices, moment by moment, and 10 seconds at a time.

The one choice we made right from those early days was that we weren't going to be doing relationship in the way this current reality does it. Right from the start, Nirmada and I acknowledged that we were creating a relationship that was beyond anything that we had ever experienced or seen. And that's how we parted ways to return to California and Australia, respectively.

NIRMADA: One of the key things to know about the journey that followed is that it was by no means straightforward. There is often a kind of 'Hollywood' expectation, when someone shares a story like ours, that there will be a happy-ever-after ending. Just because you have communion with someone doesn't mean that it's all sugar and roses.

We made an agreement with each other that anything that isn't in alignment with what is true for us, must go. We both had, and have, similar core values — to create a more conscious world everywhere we can and to have fun doing so.

We began to facilitate each other with the tools that we share throughout this book, so that we could live by those core values more and more. We created our relationship moment by moment and 10 seconds at a time. It was not about trying to make things go away or making them wrong for being there—it was more about being in non-judgment for what was showing up and clearing it when required. We use all of these tools on ourselves, every single day, and are a testimony to how well they work.

As John's marriage dissolved and we found a way to bring our lives together from opposite corners of the world, we faced a number of challenges. One of the ways we worked through those challenges was to consistently make choices in 10-second increments.

And if the choice we had made in one "10 seconds" didn't work for us, we made a different choice in the next 10 seconds, by asking: "What else is possible?" This and the other tools that we present in this book have enabled us to dismantle the existing paradigm of relationship, not only for ourselves, but also for countless others seeking a new possibility in life and relationship.

NIRMADA AND JOHN: We are choosing to be at the front of the wave—on the creative edge of what else is possible on this planet. This book is an invitation for you to join us on this wave. Just as we have both chosen to become aware of, and change, all that is disharmonious within our communion, we are here to invite you to create new possibilities in your life and relationship.

This book is about the journey and not about a final destination. And we would like to say, right from the start, that if you are looking for answers and you want to 'get it right' in relationship and stop when you get comfortable, then this probably isn't the book for you. Likewise, if you desire to hold onto your conclusions or fixed points of view, then this book is most likely not for you.

The truth is that, when we started out, neither of us could ever have imagined creating such an amazing relationship. It matched the energy of everything we'd been asking for and it didn't look like anything we had imagined. Of course, we've had moments of thinking that we didn't desire to continue our relationship, and that usually occurred when we bought other people's conclusions about what our relationship was supposed to be.

The good news was, and still is, that in the 10 seconds that followed, we knew that we could always ask: "What else is possible?" and then choose something different. And this is the gift that we would to like share with you.

As we undertake this journey together, we won't promise you that it is going to be an easy ride. However, the tools can contribute to more ease for you with whatever does show up. If you use the tools that we present in this book, moment by moment, you will learn a new way of being in relationship that will most likely make you wonder how you ever lived within the limitations of the old paradigm.

The keys to your freedom to change the limitations of relationship are here in this book, and as you practice applying these tools, you will begin to experience a level of awareness that makes it possible to expand every area of your life.

We invite you to dive into this book. You can use it as a manual for growth and change, as well as a book that you read from cover to cover. We created *Love in the Next 10 Seconds* so that you can change any area of your life and relationship by getting out of conclusions and into asking questions. The tools presented in this book are designed for creating your new paradigm in life and relationship with ease.

We wish you an infinite amount of joy and freedom as you learn to live, and love, 10 seconds at a time.

Creating Your Reality in 10-Second Increments

This book is our gift to the world and in it are tools that we have been grateful to receive from Access Consciousness, and are honored to share with you. These are the tools we use ourselves and with our clients, 10 seconds at a time, and with results that are beyond imagination. These tools and concepts contribute to your life and relationship when things are going well and they also contribute to your life and relationship when things are not going well.

If this book supports you in creating a great relationship, then we are delighted for you. If it supports you in realizing that the relationship you are in isn't working for you, then we are equally delighted for you. Either way, what we are sharing with you here will empower you to create a life and a relationship that work for you.

PART ONE

A New Paradigm
of Relationship

CHAPTER ONE

Living in 10-Second Increments

~

The Foundation for Your New Paradigm of Relationship

YOU MAY HAVE picked up this book because the title, *Love in the Next 10 Seconds,* piqued your curiosity. It suggests that you can love someone, 10 seconds at a time. At this stage, the idea of loving someone in 10-second increments might do anything from excite and thrill you, to fill you with fear about what that would actually mean for you.

Throughout this chapter, we are going to explain and illustrate the concept of how to love and make choices, 10 seconds at a time. We are going to guide you on making choices in this way, and show you how this will liberate you from the old paradigm of relationship. The tool of Making Choices in 10-Second Increments can be used in conjunction with all the other tools presented in this book and we will guide you on how to apply them to every aspect of your life.

In this chapter, we will briefly introduce additional tools that you will learn about in more detail later, laying the foundation for everything that is going to follow.

Creating Your Relationship Beyond the Commitments of the Old Paradigm

In the old paradigm of relationship, there is a familiar pattern where people often make a commitment to each other early on as to what the relationship 'should be like', and then this becomes set in stone.

Did you ever find yourself concluding what your desires, likes or dislikes were at the start of a new relationship, and then never changing or questioning these again?

Sometimes both partners start out wanting the same things. Other times, both partners desire different things, and at that point compromises are usually made. Either way, the old paradigm encourages us to design a blueprint for our relationship, which then becomes rigid and gets locked into place.

In the old paradigm of relationship, once these commitments are locked into place, it is often assumed or hoped that your partner will not change, evolve or grow. If they do change, it can be seen as some kind of violation of what you both initially agreed the relationship was supposed to be.

If growth or evolution takes place with only one partner, this can be seen by the other as a fault, a problem, or that something is wrong. Sometimes there is even blame, as the other party can bitterly proclaim, "You've changed!" as if this was somehow not expected or allowed.

How many times have you found yourself in a similar pattern, where you made a commitment to someone, assuming or hoping that neither of you was going to change? If you've been around in this cycle more than a few times and are now ready to change this, we invite you to start asking questions, such as "What else is possible?" or "What other choices are available to me?"

Throughout *Love in the Next 10 Seconds*, we will guide you, step by step, on how you can change the pattern of making conclusions about what your life and relationship are supposed to be; we will guide you on how to ask questions and make choices, 10 seconds at a time.

What if You Never Made a Wrong Choice Again?

Have you ever found yourself unable to choose something because you were afraid that you were going to make the *wrong* choice? When we show you how to make choices, 10 seconds at a time, this will begin to free you from being concerned that you will make a wrong choice.

The premise of making choices, in 10-second increments, is that if you make a choice and it doesn't work out, then you can make a new choice in the next 10 seconds. In this way, you can never make a wrong choice. You get to keep choosing every 10 seconds.

When you set something in stone, it never occurs to you that you have another choice available. The benefit of making choices, 10 seconds at a time, is that you become present in your life, because you're not trying to come to conclusions about what you are supposed to do. When you are present in your life and with your partner, you start to enjoy each moment.

Ultimately, making choices, 10 seconds at a time, gives you the freedom of choice, without needing to make yourself wrong, regardless of the outcome of what your choice creates.

The old paradigm teaches us to have the answers, rather than to ask questions and be empowered to trust our own knowing. It also teaches us to follow a set plan rather than choosing what works for us, 10 seconds at a time.

In the new paradigm, if you start planning something and it doesn't work, then you have the freedom in the next 10 seconds to make a new choice. With this freedom, you know that you have a different choice available, rather than trying to determine whether every choice that you make is either right or wrong.

AN EXERCISE TO GET YOU PRESENT WITH YOUR PARTNER

Think about your partner or someone in your life, and now love them for the next 10 seconds; that 10 seconds is over, now hate them for the next 10 seconds; that 10 seconds is over, now love them for the next 10 seconds; that 10 seconds is over, now hate them for 10 next seconds; that 10 seconds is over, now love them for the next 10 seconds. How do you feel about this person now? Better, worse or the same? We think it will actually make you feel better because you are now present with them.

This is an exercise to get you out of expectations or conclusions about what you think this person is supposed to be like.

AN EXERCISE IN BUILDING YOUR MUSCLE FOR MAKING CHOICES

You have 10 seconds to live the rest of your life, what do you choose? You have 10 seconds to live the rest of your life, now what do you choose? You have 10 seconds to live the rest of your life, now what do you choose? You have 10 seconds to live the rest of your life, now what do you choose? You have 10 seconds to live the rest of your life, now what do you choose?

How many choices did you actually come up with? Most people are not taught to keep choosing — they are just taught to choose what is 'right'.

Commitment in 10-Second Increments

The model we are presenting in *Love in the Next 10 Seconds* shows you how you can commit to your life and your relationship, 10 seconds at a time. When people hear this concept for the first time, it can often bring up concerns. We are taught that commitment gives us security. Many people believe they will be lost without a fixed commitment in relationship.

For some people, the thought of having a relationship without commitment can trigger anxiety about not being able to control their partner or their choices. And in the old paradigm, we are entrained to believe that when someone commits to us, it validates who we are. A sense of self-worth is often associated with being in a committed relationship.

We understand that commitment does work for some couples, so we are suggesting that if you choose to commit to each other, you can do so, in 10-second increments. It's possible to make commitments in 10-second increments when you are willing to let go of your expectations and projections about what you thought commitments were supposed to be.

In this chapter, and throughout this book, we are going to support you in moving beyond any concerns you may have about creating your relationship in 10-second increments. We will be sharing a number of tools with you that will allow this transition to unfold for you with ease. In this new model, you can continue to make life choices that might *seem* like they are fixed commitments — such as buying a house together, building a business together, and so on.

However, the difference is that you will also learn to be prepared to let them go if they are not working for you. When you are willing to lose anything that is not working for you, this gives you the freedom of choice. This doesn't mean that you actually have to lose anything, just that you have the *willingness* to lose anything, in order to not be controlled by any fixed points of view or fixed commitments. The willingness to lose anything, in this way, allows for new possibilities to show up in every 10 seconds.

Many Eastern traditions have taught the concept of non-attachment. Though this can often seem like a nice concept to apply to our lives and relationships, the average person in the West just doesn't know how to do this. However, when you start living in 10-second increments, you experience non-attachment while continuing to create, build and actualize things with your partner.

TWELVE TOOLS THAT ALLOW YOU TO PRACTICE MAKING CHOICES IN 10-SECOND INCREMENTS

(We introduce them here, and we will explore them more deeply later on in the book.)

1. Choosing in 10-Second Increments

The basic premise of this tool is that you can make choices for anything in your life, 10 seconds at a time. For example, you can choose to be with your partner, 10 seconds at a time, until you don't desire to choose that anymore. How liberating is this, compared to: "I have made a commitment to my partner and therefore I have to stick with them for the rest of my life."

When you make choices in 10-second increments, some of the relationship issues from the old paradigm can be eliminated, such as expecting your partner to behave a certain way and then getting upset when they don't. You no longer try to control the choices of your partner and you learn to have allowance for the choices they make, 10 seconds at a time.

One of the first questions this evokes is: "Doesn't this just mean that they will do whatever they please?" It can be unsettling for some people to set their partner free in this way, and to not be thinking in terms of possession and control.

However, we also include something known as the "Kingdom of We" in this choice. That means both partners have an awareness of the other, and an understanding of what is basically going to work for one another. If both partners were coming from the "Kingdom of Me" and had little consideration and awareness of their partner, then admittedly, making choices in 10-second increments could feel a bit like a 'free for all'.

What we are presenting here is very different from the concept of 'free love', which has its own set of conclusions. When you make choices in your relationship, 10 seconds at a time and from the "Kingdom of We", you also include the awareness of your partner in the choices that you make.

AN EXERCISE FOR LEARNING HOW TO MAKE CHOICES IN 10-SECOND INCREMENTS

- For 3 minutes, choose to do something different every 10 seconds.

- For example, you might choose to go outside and smell the flowers, then pet the dog, then go inside, then send a text to your lover and so on.

2. Fighting in 10-Second Increments

Have you ever had a fight with your partner that lasted hours, days or even weeks? How many hours of your life have you spent fighting in your current or previous relationships? How often have you wished to find a way of ending a fight, but you never really knew how?

When making choices in 10-second increments, you can choose to fight in one 10 seconds and then you can choose something different in the next 10 seconds.

This may actually require more than 10 seconds to implement, especially if both of you are triggered. However, the basic premise is that if you are fighting, you can simply just pause and ask your partner: "What other choices are available to us in the next 10 seconds?" or "What's *really* going on here?" Sometimes asking questions like these can interrupt the pattern of the fight and then you have the next 10 seconds to make a new choice.

You can practice Making Choices in 10-Second Increments when you are not in 'fight mode', so that you can implement it more easily when you are fighting.

3. Letting Go of Significance and Relevance in 10-Second Increments

In the old paradigm of relationship, many of us have been entrained to make everything significant and relevant. If a partner forgets a birthday or an anniversary, we have learned to make it mean that they don't love or care about us. The list of things 'significant and relevant' goes on, as in whether your partner has texted you or not, called you or not, wants to spend time with you or not, says or does the 'right thing' or not, and so on. How many of us have made our partner's choices and actions significant and relevant and then concluded that it meant something about us, or how they felt about us?

In the new paradigm of Making Choices in 10-Second Increments, we encourage you to get out of the habit of making everything significant and relevant. When you learn how to let go of needing things to be significant and relevant in your relationship, your partner's actions and behaviors are then simply seen as an interesting choice they are making in that 10 seconds, rather than a reflection on you.

How many of your past arguments in relationship have been a result of needing to make things significant and relevant? If you find yourself arguing in one 10 seconds, you can ask yourself in the next 10 seconds, "Is this really relevant?"

JOHN: Have you noticed how easily kids let go of things? I noticed this with my own children when they were young. They would misbehave in some way, and I would get mad at them. After about five minutes they would let it go, as though nothing had occurred.

What if we could all have this same kind of ease with letting go of disagreements in relationship, 10 seconds at a time?

---

4. Letting Go of Judgment in 10-Second Increments

Judgment has become an integral part of the way we function in the old paradigm of relationship and is used as a way of controlling others out of choice. Many people are taught to have fixed points of view about who they think their partner should be, and then judge them if they don't conform or live up to those expectations.

How many times have you found yourself in the pattern of making your partner wrong so that you could be right? What if you no longer had to judge the 'rightness' or the 'wrongness' of the choices that you or your partner are making?

When many couples argue, they often find themselves trying to be the winner in order not to be the loser. For one partner to win and the other to lose, judgment is always required. When you stop having the need to judge if you, or your partner, are the winner or the loser, then everything in your relationship becomes just a choice.

In the new paradigm, when you learn how to make choices in 10-second increments, and you also have allowance for the choices that your partner makes in 10-second increments, you begin to function beyond the limitations of judgment.

We are often taught to judge everything as 'right or wrong' or 'good or bad'. This may seem like we have a choice; however, it's really a choice created from a conclusion about what is right or wrong and not from asking questions. Learning to ask questions is a way to practice getting out of judgment and into making choices 10 seconds at a time. We will be exploring how to do this further in Chapter 3.

5. Gifting and Receiving in 10-Second Increments

In the new paradigm, we use the term "gifting and receiv-ing", rather than 'giving and taking', as it is less about the exchange of objects and more about the way that you can show up with your partner, in each 10 seconds.

In the old paradigm, the concept of giving and taking is commonly used. Give and take in *this* way is often played like a game of push and pull. Oftentimes this game is played with little understanding of what the other person actually wants.

Have you ever tried giving your partner something that they didn't ask for or desire? How was it received? Or maybe there was a time you were given something that you didn't want and then you were expected to give your partner something in return?

Oftentimes when there is tension or friction in the rela-tionship, one or both partners tend to withdraw from the act of gifting and receiving with the other. In con-trast, in the new paradigm, gifting and receiving is not dependent upon whether you think the relationship is 'going well' or not. You continue gifting and receiving with your partner, 10 seconds at a time, when there is conflict, as well as when things are going well.

An example of gifting to your partner when they are upset is: ask your partner if you can touch their body and if they say 'yes', you can, for instance, put your hands on the center of their chest or their back and contribute to them energetically.

NIRMADA: Even if we are upset with one another, we still place our hands on each other. The other person receives it almost every time. Sometimes, one of us just needs space too. Part of gifting and receiving is also being able to allow your partner to have space when needed.

---

6. Making Love in 10-Second Increments!

You may wonder if we are joking, when we say that we make love in 10-second increments. Your initial reaction might be to laugh and say that this is a step too far, especially if you have learned that the performance aspect of making love is significant.

In the old paradigm, if sex has been a 'good performance' then both parties often feel satisfied and there is a sense of achievement. On an 'off-day', however, one or both parties may go into judgment about themselves or their partner, if it hasn't gone as expected.

In the old paradigm, we are taught that everything about lovemaking is supposed to be significant and meaningful. In heterosexual relationships, it matters if the man gets an erection. If he doesn't, or if he loses his erection mid-performance, the woman often makes it mean something about her. And it matters if the woman has an orgasm or not. If she doesn't, the man often makes it mean something about him. The length of the performance of lovemaking also matters. Many of us have learned to attach meaning and significance to what occurs and what doesn't occur during lovemaking.

What if you didn't have to dance this tired old dance anymore? What if you could enjoy making love, 10 seconds at a time? In our relationship, when we make love, one moment we can be hot and heavy, and 10 seconds later, one or both of us can choose something different. There is no obligation to complete what we started. Also, we can be in the middle of a task, and we will suddenly choose to throw our clothes off and start having fun.

This makes lovemaking so light and easy for us. How much more ease and fun would it be for you if you were to take the performance element out of sex? What about if you also took the judgment out of it? When you let go of the 'we've started so we have to finish' idea, you open yourself up to a tremendously freeing way of gifting and receiving with your partner, 10 seconds at a time.

We would like to invite you to change the box of relationship that says: "I can only enjoy lovemaking under these conditions," and "I can't enjoy lovemaking under those conditions." What if *you* could choose to enjoy lovemaking, 10 seconds at a time?

7. Choosing Consciousness in 10-Second Increments

Love in the Next 10 Seconds was created to empower you to become more conscious and aware in your life and relationship. Part of having a conscious relationship is being able to recognize when you have 'fallen asleep at the wheel', or in other words, become unconscious.

Unconsciousness often occurs when we cut off awareness and allow our learned behaviors and programs to take over. If you have a moment of unconsciousness in your relationship, you can ask: "What 10 seconds of unconsciousness did I have that created this?" Asking this question can bring you back to the present moment—it creates more awareness and clarity.

Remember, if you choose something in one 10 seconds and it doesn't work for you, you can choose something else in the next 10 seconds. If you recognize that you have made an unconscious choice, you can always ask, "What other choices are available?" in the next 10 seconds. Asking questions in this way leads to new choices, which lead to new possibilities for your life and your relationship.

8. Un-creating Problems in 10-Second Increments

In this book we are going to show you how many of the problems experienced in life and relationship are often inventions created from our fixed points of view. Once you become aware that many of these so-called problems are actually inventions, this book will guide you on how to un-create them, 10 seconds at a time.

When you recognize that you have invented a problem, you can change it by asking questions. A question you can ask is: "What invention am I using to create the problem I am choosing?" We suggest that you continue asking this question until you notice that the energy has changed.

Remember, if you have invented a problem in one 10 seconds, you can choose to un-create it in the next 10 seconds. We will be discussing this in more detail later in the book.

NIRMADA: When our relationship started, John was still working in the mines in Australia. He started work at 6 a.m., so we would speak daily at his 5 a.m. One day he didn't pick up the phone when I called him at 5 a.m. and I didn't hear from him until 7 a.m. During those two hours, I began telling myself stories like "He did it on purpose," and "He doesn't want to speak to me anymore."

I was so convinced my stories were real that I was sure I had been dissed. At 7 a.m. I received a text from John saying that his phone battery had died overnight causing him to be an hour late for work as he had no alarm to wake him up. I realized in that moment that the entire situation was an invented problem that didn't actually exist. And in hindsight, it seemed quite absurd, since as long as I had known John, he had always been true to his word every time we scheduled anything together.

9. Asking "Who Does This Belong To?" in 10-Second Increments

Asking the questions "Who does this belong to?" or "Is this really mine?" are tools we will guide you on how to use for changing things when you are feeling stuck or when you realize that you are not being yourself.

Have you ever had an experience where you felt like you were behaving in a way that didn't seem like you? If this occurs, you can ask: "Who does this belong to?" or "Is this really mine?" These questions and concepts at first sound strange to many people because they are not logical or cognitive in the way they work. We invite you to see for yourself how using these questions can change many things for you and your body.

NIRMADA: One day, John was feeling stuck, heavy, and concerned about money. I asked him, "Is this really your point of view?" and he replied, "No!" and started laughing. If after asking this question, the stuck energy gets lighter for the person or goes away altogether, this is an indication that the concern or upset was never really theirs in the first place.

JOHN: One night I woke up with a really bad headache. After tossing for some time, I finally asked the question, "Who does this belong to?" and immediately the pain lightened up and then went away altogether. I started telling Nirmada that I was having the thought in my head that it wasn't possible to change something like this so quickly and easily. She said: "That's an interesting thought you are having—who does that belong to?" and then the thought went away. This was an indication that the headache and the thoughts associated with it were never mine to begin with.

Within 10 seconds of having an upset or being out of sorts, you can ask: "Who does this belong to?" or "Is this really mine?" If, when asking these questions, you notice things changing and the heaviness getting lighter, you may find that many of what you assumed were your own thoughts, feelings and emotions were actually adopted by you and not really yours.

When you realize the upset is something that you have adopted and that it doesn't truly belong to you, it often loses its power over you. Once you recognize it isn't actually yours, you can make a new choice beyond the upset, in the next 10 seconds.

The tools of "Who Does This Belong To?" and "Is This Really Mine?" will be discussed in more detail in Chapter 5.

10. Nurturing the Body in 10-Second Increments

Nurturing your partner's body is a powerful way for you to connect in your relationship. The body is a sensory awareness organism, and being aware of what your body and your partner's body require, in each 10 seconds, opens you both up to receiving more. When the body is ignored, it can lead to disharmony and a sense of separation from yourself or your partner.

One way to connect with your own body is to ask: "Body, is there anything you require in this 10 seconds?" and allow yourself to receive the awareness and information that your body is giving you. Additional questions you can ask are: "Body, what would you like to eat?" or "Body, what clothes would you like to wear today?" or "Body, what would be something fun to do in the next 10 seconds?"

Asking questions in this way can contribute to having more harmony and ease with your body. When you are aware that your partner's body would benefit from some nurturing, you can ask them: "Is there anything that I can contribute to your body in the next 10 seconds?" You may find that when you ask this question, your hands naturally rest somewhere upon your partner.

JOHN: When I sense that Nirmada's body requires a contribution from me, I simply ask, "What energy can I contribute to Nirmada's body in the next 10 seconds?" I then lay my hands on her body wherever they are drawn to go.

NIRMADA: Sometimes John naturally puts his hands on my body and other times I will ask him, "Could you contribute something to my body right now?"

In the new paradigm, when things are going well with your partner, you can nurture and contribute to their body. When things are not going so well, you can also nurture and contribute to their body to allow the situation to change. You may notice how different this is from the old paradigm, where intimacy is often withheld when things aren't going well in the relationship.

11. Expanding your Allowance in 10-Second Increments

Another key tool that we share in this book is learning to expand your allowance. Expanding your allowance creates more harmony and ease with yourself and your partner. When you learn to have allowance for the choices that your partner makes, even if they don't make sense to you in the moment, it allows for both of you to live and love, 10 seconds at a time.

Having allowance in this way is different from just tolerating anything. Tolerating things requires judgment of what's 'right or wrong' or 'good or bad', and therefore eliminates making choices in 10-second increments. Expanding your allowance includes allowing your partner to choose the things that *they* desire to change. This is very different from having expectations that they should change the things that you think they should.

If your partner is having an upset, then you can choose to expand your allowance for what is occurring. Expanding your allowance in situations like this includes remembering that it may be an invented problem or upset that your partner believes is real.

JOHN: When I can see that Nirmada is on edge, I expand my allowance, rather than getting caught up in the fact that she is upset. This allows me to ask her questions, such as "Is there anything I can contribute to you in the next 10 seconds?" or "Do you need to expand your allowance right now?" This contributes to both of us having more harmony and ease.

To get your allowance to expand, you simply *ask* for it to expand. We explain this in more detail in Chapter 2.

12. Practicing Acknowledgment
in 10-Second Increments

Acknowledgment is a tool that you can use with your partner when things are going well and when things are challenging.

When you acknowledge what is going well, it allows for more of the good things to show up. Acknowledgment allows you to recognize and increase that which is working well; also, it reminds you that a different choice is available in the next 10 seconds, when things aren't going well.

- What are three things you can acknowledge about yourself?
- What are three things you can acknowledge about your partner?

We use the tool of Acknowledgment on a daily basis in creating our lives and our relationship, 10 seconds at a time. We also use it often with the other people in our lives.

NIRMADA: John and I use the tool of Acknowledgment to change the energy of an argument in order to create more ease. In one 10 seconds we could be bickering and in the next 10 seconds we could choose to acknowledge each other for three things we are grateful for about one another. After acknowledging each other in this way, the argument dissipates. We then move on to creating something new in the next 10 seconds.

Summary of the Tools, Concepts and Questions from Chapter One

1. "What other choices are available?" in the next 10 seconds and "What's really going on here?" — Questions you can ask to create new possibilities when there are challenges.

2. "What else is possible?"® — A question you can ask to create greater possibilities when things are going well and when things are not going well.

3. "What 10 seconds of unconsciousness did I have that created this?" — A question designed to help you become more aware, when you have 'fallen asleep at the wheel' and had a moment of unconsciousness.

4. Twelve tools which allow you to practice Making Choices in 10-Second Increments:

   1. Choosing in 10-Second Increments
   2. Fighting in 10-Second Increments
   3. Letting Go of Significance and Relevance in 10-Second Increments
   4. Letting Go of Judgment in 10-Second Increments
   5. Gifting and Receiving in 10-Second Increments
   6. Making Love in 10-Second Increments!
   7. Choosing Consciousness in 10-Second Increments
   8. Un-creating Problems in 10-Second Increments
   9. Asking "Who Does This Belong To?"® in 10-Second Increments
   10. Nurturing the Body in 10-Second Increments
   11. Expanding your Allowance in 10-Second Increments
   12. Practicing Acknowledgment in 10-Second Increments

Learning to make choices in 10-second increments is really about understanding that choice is always available. Once you choose to no longer operate from fixed points of view, judgments or conclusions, you open yourself up to new possibilities in every moment.

We'll explore the tool of Making Choices in 10-Second Increments in more detail as the book unfolds. We will also look in more depth at each of the tools that we have outlined briefly in this chapter.

In the next chapter, we'll begin looking at The Five Elements of Intimacy, and how you can use them, alongside the other tools, to create more harmony and a deeper connection with yourself and your partner.

CHAPTER TWO

The Five Elements
of Intimacy

~

HONOR • TRUST • VULNERABILITY
ALLOWANCE • GRATITUDE

MAKING CHOICES IN 10-Second Increments is fundamental to the new paradigm of relationship, and **The Five Elements of Intimacy** form the foundation upon which this new model is built.

The Five Elements of Intimacy are Honor, Trust, Vulnerability, Allowance and Gratitude. Each one of these elements complements the others, and when all five elements are present in your relationship, it can seem effortless, even when there are challenges.

Living The Five Elements of Intimacy

In order to be able to live The Five Elements of Intimacy with another, it is essential to experience them first and foremost with yourself.

JOHN: When Nirmada and I first met, we had a level of ease and joy together that was effortless. As our relationship unfolded, we realized that one of the things that contributed to it working so well was that, together, we had a harmony with all of The Five Elements of Intimacy.

Honor

The first element of The Five Elements of Intimacy is Honor. In the new paradigm of relationship, to honor your partner is to treat them, and yourself, with regard. This includes honoring what works for your partner, and at the same time, honoring what works for you. When you honor yourself and your choices, you stand by them, even if others don't approve.

Honoring your partner is allowing them to choose what works for them, and not expecting them to do what you want them to do.

In the new paradigm of relationship, honor is not just something that you commit to once, as in the traditional wedding vows. Instead, honoring is something that you choose to do moment by moment and 10 seconds at a time. This means that honoring becomes something that you practice with yourself and your partner. Honor builds up over time as you continue to practice honoring yourself and your partner on a daily basis.

NIRMADA: On one occasion, I asked John if he wanted to have sex and he said, "No." I could have gone into the wrongness of me, or into the judgment of him. Instead, I just honored his choice. Later, John revealed that he hadn't been feeling well. His choice to not have sex with me in that 10 seconds had nothing to do with me. I didn't make his choice personal or significant, and that allowed for the situation to unfold; when John was feeling better he naturally became more intimate with me.

If you desire to have sex and your partner doesn't, what would it take for you to honor each of your choices without going into wrongness or judgment? Judgment has become a normalized way of functioning in the old paradigm of relationship.

How much have we all been entrained to dishonor ourselves, and each other, by judging one another? Recognizing when you have gone into judgment, and then making a different choice, is one of the ways of honoring yourself and others in your life.

When you find yourself going into judgment, you can ask: "Who does this judgment belong to?" or "Is this judgment really mine?" (This is a tool we will explore further in Chapter 5.)

Honoring is not about cutting off your awareness to tolerate things that aren't working for you, although many of us have been taught to function this way. When we make a conclusion like 'I love you, so therefore I am going to stay with you,' there can be a tendency to cut off our awareness in order to tolerate things that don't actually work for us.

Anytime we conclude in this way, it can be a dishonoring of ourselves. When we are honoring of ourselves, we start to become more aware and this allows us to know what does and doesn't work for us.

Honoring is also not about being artificially 'nice' to your partner. Being 'nice' to your partner, while secretly going along with something that doesn't work for you, can be dishonoring to both of you. Treating your partner with regard requires you to be honest with them and honest with yourself.

This includes being honest about what works for you and what doesn't work for you. Sometimes expressing what's true for you can be confronting to your partner. If you are able to express what is true for you without going into judgment, it's an honoring of both of you.

Honoring your partner is also acknowledging where they are currently functioning from. Have you ever found yourself feeling frustrated when your partner doesn't show up in a way that you perceived they could? You may be able to see there is something greater they could choose and they are not currently choosing it. Perhaps they are not ready to show up in the way that you know is possible.

Honoring your partner is treating them with enough regard to recognize what they are capable of choosing or not capable of choosing. Honoring yourself is knowing that you also have choice, 10 seconds at a time. The tools contained in this book will assist you in navigating your way through having allowance for yourself and your partner, and honoring the choices that both of you make.

By asking questions, such as "What else is possible?" or "What other choices are available?", you can start to develop the practice of honoring yourself and your partner.

NIRMADA: When John and I first got together, we were in very different living, working and family situations. John was in a job that was no longer a match for him. I could see the possibility that he could choose something greater than he was choosing. I asked him a lot of questions so he could become empowered to receive this awareness for himself. He began choosing what worked for him by leaving his job, changing his living situation and starting new creative ventures. Being aware of what he could receive 10 seconds at a time, and honoring him where he was at, allowed for new possibilities to show up for both of us, and for our relationship.

Questions to practice honoring yourself and your partner:

- "Am I treating myself with regard and honoring what is true for me?"

- "Am I treating my partner with regard and honoring their choices?"

Trust

The second element of The Five Elements of Intimacy is Trust. Trust in the new paradigm of relationship is based on using your awareness to know what's true for you, 10 seconds at a time. What's true for you in this 10 seconds may not be true for you in the next 10 seconds.

Trust in the old paradigm of relationship is more akin to blind faith. Saying something along the lines of 'I trust that my partner will never hurt me' is not really trust—it is more like having blind faith and being obliged to follow what you have concluded or believed to be true, rather than being aware of what *is* true, 10 seconds at a time.

What commonly occurs at the start of a new relationship is that each partner must earn the trust of the other. There can also be a series of 'tests' that either party has to pass in order to prove that they are trustworthy. People often look for the 'rightness' or the 'wrongness' of their partner's choices. Once we have concluded what we believe to be right or wrong about our partner, we then start to cut off our awareness of anything that doesn't match those conclusions.

In the new paradigm, trust is based on trusting your own awareness. It is very different from collecting evidence about whether or not your partner can be trusted, or placing blind faith in them. The basis of trust in The Five Elements of Intimacy is that you trust that your partner is going to do what they are *going* to do.

What if you could stop trying to figure out or control what you think your partner should do and instead, have allowance for what they *actually* choose. Having allowance for the choices that you and your partner make is empowering and creates more harmony and ease in your relationship.

JOHN: I've asked my teenage kids many times in the past to clean up after themselves in the kitchen; however, they still leave a mess. By trusting they are going to do what they are going to do, it creates more harmony and ease for all of us.

Many people have learned to cut off their awareness in a relationship and then they stop trusting themselves. How many relationships have started where the person knew in advance it wasn't going to work and they went ahead with it anyway?

JOHN: As I highlighted earlier, one way to start building trust in your own awareness is, before you have sex with somebody for the first time, you can ask these four questions:

- "If I have sex with this person, will it be fun?"

- "If I have sex with this person, will it be easy?"

- "If I have sex with this person, will I learn something?"

- "If I have sex with this person, will they be grateful?"

As I mentioned earlier, before I met Nirmada, I had asked myself these four questions about many women. When I met Nirmada, it was the first time I got a light and expansive response to all four questions. I had built up a deep trust with my own awareness by asking these questions, and choosing to not have sex with anyone until all four responses to these questions were light and expansive for me.

By trusting my own awareness of what was true for me, it made the choice easy to have sex with Nirmada. (We will talk more about how to perceive if something is light or heavy for you in Chapter 4.)

By learning to ask questions, you can practice trusting your own awareness to choose what works for you.

Here are some questions to practice trusting your own awareness:

- "Am I trusting my own awareness?"

- "What could I be or do today to have more awareness right away?"

- "Am I trusting my partner to do what they are going to do, regardless of what I think they should do?"

When you ask questions in this way, it creates an opening for you to receive more awareness. Remember, you are not looking for an answer here, and the awareness from asking questions will come to you...when it does.

Vulnerability

The third element of The Five Elements of Intimacy is Vulnerability. In the new paradigm of relationship, vulnerability is regarded as a strength, and it creates more intimacy with yourself and your partner. In the old paradigm, vulnerability is often considered a weakness.

Oftentimes people put up their barriers as a protective mechanism against being hurt by judgment or ridicule, rather than allowing themselves to be vulnerable.

Many people learn to carefully calculate the person or situation in front of them and only then decide if it's safe enough to open up and be themselves. As children, when we were yelled at or made wrong when saying what was true for us, many of us learned to put up barriers in order to feel safe.

Putting up barriers creates separation, cuts off your awareness and ultimately limits your receiving. You may have even stopped being who you are naturally, as you made other people's judgments more valuable than your own awareness of what is true for you.

As the subtitle of this book, "Living Without Limits", suggests, we are encouraging you every step of the way to be empowered to be all of you and to know that you have choice, 10 seconds at a time.

In the old paradigm of relationship, one interpretation of vulnerability might have been allowing yourself to be stepped on. In the new paradigm, vulnerability is about lowering your barriers and receiving things without needing them to be 'right or wrong' or 'good or bad'.

True receiving, in this sense, is about receiving more awareness. The more awareness you have, the more possibilities and choices become available to you. In the old paradigm, putting up barriers was judged necessary for protection. In the new paradigm, your only true protection is your ability to be aware and to trust your own knowing.

Becoming more aware can be uncomfortable as you start to see and perceive things that you had previously avoided. Lowering your barriers and allowing yourself to be vulnerable can sometimes feel as though you are being rubbed 'raw'. Although it's not always comfortable, being vulnerable will create more intimacy and connectedness with your partner.

JOHN: Here is one of the ways I use vulnerability with Nirmada. If she has an upset, rather than trying to 'do the man thing' and fix the situation, I lower my barriers, and receive her and the situation without a point of view. This creates more harmony and ease and usually allows whatever is occurring to dissipate. This also empowers Nirmada to use her own awareness to change the situation.

There are many examples in popular culture of people who have been able to maintain their inner strength while also being vulnerable. Oprah Winfrey is a prime example of this. Think about Oprah for a moment. What is it that makes people relate to her? She is very upfront about growing up poor, and having many life challenges. However, she uses her challenges to connect with her audience. This level of vulnerability is at the heart of her popularity.

NIRMADA: When I first met John, we naturally had a level of vulnerability and presence with each other, which was sometimes uncomfortable. We didn't try to cover up who we were or figure out what we thought we should be for the other person. As a result, we have created an intimacy with each other without an agenda or a fixed point of view of how our relationship should be.

This allows for us to have a deeper sense of harmony and connection with each other, without the need to put up barriers.

If you are in allowance of your partner, and you are not judging them, it then becomes easier for you to be more vulnerable with them. However, if there is a lot of judgment and both of you are defending your points of view, then learning to create a relationship beyond judgment will increase your intimacy with each other. We will explore how to create a relationship beyond judgment in Chapter 6.

AN EXERCISE TO PRACTICE LOWERING YOUR BARRIERS

You don't have to know cognitively how to lower your barriers, you simply just energetically ask for your barriers to lower and intend for them to lower. You can practice this on your own or with your partner. If at first this seems unfamiliar, we suggest you keep practicing and notice what changes. Whenever you notice a new barrier coming up, in the next 10 seconds you can choose to tell yourself: "I'm not going there!" and then push it down.

Questions to ask to have more vulnerability:

- "Do I have barriers up right now?"

- "Am I being vulnerable right now?"

- "Do I have barriers up to receiving right now?"

Allowance

Allowance is the fourth element of The Five Elements of Intimacy. Practicing allowance enables you to get out of making conclusions about what your relationship is supposed to be, and allows you to create it 10 seconds at a time, with harmony and ease.

If you have allowance for yourself, no matter what shows up, then you can also have allowance for others. What if you could have allowance for yourself *and* for your partner without the need to exclude or reject anything about either one of you?

Many of us, under the influence of the old paradigm, have been entrained to control our partners so they don't do anything that violates what we have already concluded is, or isn't, allowed. If you are not in allowance of your partner and have a preconceived idea of who you think they should be, this ends up creating limitations and what we call "The Box of Relationship".

In the new paradigm, you practice having allowance for the things that your partner says or does, rather than judging them or making them wrong. We will show you how you can learn to do this by using Interesting Point of View, a tool that we will be exploring in Chapter 3.

When your partner has points of view that are different from yours, you may have learned to either resist and react to, or align and agree with, those points of view. Arguments in relationship are often based on fixed points of view about what we have concluded is right or wrong, good or bad. From this place, we think the conclusions we have made are the *only* choices we have. In most cases, these fixed points of view have been handed down to us, and we adopted them and live with them as though they were our own.

The new possibility we are bringing forth in this book is for you to learn to be in allowance of what your partner says or does, without having a point of view about it being right or wrong. When you don't have a belief that anything is right or wrong, you then *just* have choice.

Allowance in 10-Second Increments

The tools of Allowance and Making Choices in 10-Second Increments are complementary to one other. The more allowance you have, the easier it will become for you to make choices in 10-second increments.

If you chose to create your life and relationship 10 seconds at a time, would there be a need to control your partner? We suggest you practice having allowance for the choices that you and your partner make, beyond judging whether you think those choices are 'good or bad' or 'right or wrong'.

A reminder: When you choose something and it works, you can choose it again. And, if you choose something and it doesn't work, you can choose something new in the next 10 seconds.

Allowance and Awareness

When we speak about allowance, we are not suggesting that you become a doormat or just tolerate anything your partner says or does. In the old paradigm, many people have learned to make things easier by not 'rocking the boat'. Oftentimes, they cut off their awareness in order to tolerate things that don't actually work for them. Without having allowance for your partner, eventually you may find yourself reacting or putting up barriers as a result of tolerating too many things that haven't worked for you.

Rather than cutting off your awareness in order to tolerate your partner's actions, you can instead expand your allowance, while simultaneously being aware of what works for you. The more your awareness increases, the more important it will become for you to expand your allowance.

As previously highlighted in this chapter, as you become more aware, it can get uncomfortable. When you expand your allowance, you create more ease and comfort with having more awareness.

To expand your allowance, you simply ask for your allowance to expand. You don't have to know how it works, just ask and your allowance will expand.

For example, if you are irritated by your partner's actions, rather than reacting to them, you can instead ask for your allowance to expand.

The tools presented in this book encourage you to be empowered by knowing what works for you and to be able to say things to your partner, such as "I'm sorry, that's not going to work for me" or "What's going to work for me is _____."

Knowing what isn't going to work for you is different from rejecting your partner for who they are. It's more about you choosing what you know works for you, 10 seconds at a time, and also having allowance for the choices that you and your partner make.

Allowance and The Kingdom of We

Allowance and The Kingdom of We work well together. If we only make choices for what is good for ourselves, then we are operating from The Kingdom of Me, and are not being inclusive of our partner. When we expand our awareness and choices to include what is good for ourselves and our partner, then we are making choices based on The Kingdom of We.

When you give up your points of view about needing things to be 'right or wrong' or 'good or bad', and instead you are in allowance, you create more harmony and ease in your life and relationship. Remember, it's easier to have allowance for your partner when you also have allowance for yourself.

Oftentimes things do not show up as we have imagined. We invite you to practice having allowance for things showing up as they do. And when you do this, you allow the possibility for things to show up greater than you have imagined.

Allowance for Where Your Partner is Now

We invite you to be in allowance for exactly where your partner is right now. Many people choose a relationship based on a future vision of who they think their partner will become. In the new paradigm, you practice seeing the potential of your partner, and at the same time you practice being in allowance of where they are right now.

This means you have trust and allowance that your partner will change and grow at their *own* pace. This includes having allowance for things to unfold in layers, rather than trying to push them along.

You can be open to the possibility that at any moment, anything can show up in your life and relationship. However, just because you know that it can show up, doesn't mean it is going to show up right now, or that it will show up in the future. The new paradigm encourages you to be aware of possibilities and simultaneously to have allowance for 'what is'.

Having allowance for where your partner is now also includes being in allowance for what they choose. In the new model that we are presenting here, even though it might seem as though you know a 'better way', you choose to not push that on your partner. We encourage you to ask questions of yourself and your partner, and as a result of this, you will both get your own awareness...when you get it.

JOHN: When Nirmada and I would go on a trip together, she used to take a long time to pack and spread her things all over the house. I saw that there was an easier way to do it. However, rather than telling her how she should do it, I chose to be in allowance instead. By allowing her to receive her own awareness of what could work better, she started to naturally change. It used to take her a few days to pack, and now it only takes her a few hours.

NIRMADA: When I first met John, I had much more exposure to the tools that we are sharing with you in this book. Sometimes I could see the possibilities for what else he could choose, long before he could. However, I practiced having allowance for where he was at, without pushing him on what he could choose. Ultimately, this allowed him to become more aware for creating something greater for himself.

A reminder: A choice is only good for 10 seconds. If the choice you make in this 10 seconds doesn't work, rather than going into wrongness, you can make a new choice in the next 10 seconds. This allows you and your partner to show up as you are in each moment and to begin your adventure together in living without limits.

Questions for expanding your allowance:

- "Am I having allowance for myself?"

- "Am I having allowance for my partner?"

- "Does my allowance require expanding?"

Gratitude

The fifth element of The Five Elements of Intimacy is Gratitude. Gratitude is a tool that you can practice using with yourself as well as with your partner. In the new paradigm, gratitude is an integral part of the relationship—you are not just grateful for what your partner does or says, you are grateful for who they are.

When things are going well in your relationship, gratitude can be used to expand this energy. When things are not going well in your relationship, gratitude can be used to change the energy and create more harmony and ease.

If you and your partner are in an argument, one example of a way you can use gratitude to change the energy is to take a breather and ask: "What are three things that we are each grateful for?" Sometimes it may be easy to say three things that you are grateful for about your partner, and other times it may be easier to express your gratitude in more general terms.

We ourselves have quickly and easily resolved many arguments by taking a pause and saying three things we are grateful for. More often than not, this dissipates the argument and then we move on to something else in the next 10 seconds.

Gratitude and Judgment

Whenever you are being grateful, it is impossible for you to be in judgment at the same time. In the new paradigm, gratitude is used as a tool to change situations and it helps you to get out of judging anything as 'right or wrong' or 'good or bad'.

In the old paradigm, many of us were taught to withdraw our gratitude for our partner if they did something we didn't like. In the new paradigm, gratitude can be used on a daily basis, and is not withdrawn if your partner is having an off-day or there is an upset.

Non-Verbal Gratitude

Gratitude can be verbally expressed as well as energetically. Sometimes saying what you are grateful for to your partner is what they require. And sometimes "being the energy" of gratitude with your partner is what they require.

NIRMADA: In the beginning of our relationship, I perceived that I wasn't being appreciated by John, as he didn't always verbally express his gratitude for me. After some discussion, we realized that John would often "be the energy" of gratitude with me and not necessarily verbalize it.

John has learned to express his gratitude verbally to me as well as energetically. I have learned to receive the energy of John being grateful as well as hearing it verbally from him. Through this journey we have both expanded our capacity to gift to each other, and receive gratitude from each other, in many different ways.

Gratitude and Acknowledgment

Have you ever noticed how much you thrive when you receive gratitude and acknowledgment? Have you ever noticed how much your partner thrives when they receive gratitude and acknowledgment?

In the old paradigm, when you first start a new relationship, you are grateful for everything the person says or does. Then, after the 'honeymoon' period is over, you start to function in a different away. Expectations, projections and conclusions can gradually slip in and push gratitude aside.

Remember, gratitude and acknowledgment are always available to use for creating more harmony and ease with your partner.

Genuine gratitude is much more than just empty praise. It is a way of being with your partner that allows you to contribute to them without judgment. When you are grateful for your partner and who they are, you naturally find yourself acknowledging the things that you recognize and admire in them.

Some examples of how you can express gratitude are: "I would like to acknowledge the way you handled that situation," or "I'm really grateful for your contribution to me!"

If you aren't already doing so, we invite you to practice expressing gratitude for yourself and your partner on a daily basis. You can express gratitude for anything in your life, whether it's something small *or* something big.

Masaru Emoto was a Japanese author and researcher whose work was centered around the effect that consciousness has on the molecular structure of water. His studies show what happens to water when you say hateful things around it, as opposed to what happens to it when you say loving and kind things. The molecular structure of the water changes according to the energy that gets projected upon it. Under a microscope, the structure of water, when you say loving and grateful things to it, looks something like a beautiful snowflake, and if you say hateful things around water, it loses its pattern. Our bodies are mainly comprised of water, so can you perceive how using gratitude and acknowledgment would positively affect the molecular structure of our bodies?

Questions to practice using gratitude and acknowledgment:

- "What am I grateful for about myself today?"

- "What am I grateful for about my partner today?"

- "What can I acknowledge about myself today?"

- "What can I acknowledge about my partner today?"

Summary of the Tools, Concepts and Questions from Chapter Two

1. The Five Elements of Intimacy are the foundation upon which the new paradigm of relationship is built. They are:

    *   **Honor:** When you honor your partner, you are treating them, and yourself, with regard.

    *   **Trust:** Trust means trusting your own awareness and trusting that your partner is going to do what they are going to do.

    *   **Vulnerability:** Vulnerability means not putting up barriers to your partner and receiving them as they are.

    *   **Allowance**: Practicing allowance enables you to get out of making conclusions about what your relationship is supposed to be, and allows you to create it 10 seconds at a time, with harmony and ease.

    *   **Gratitude**: Gratitude is an integral part of the relationship: you are not just grateful for what your partner does or says, you are grateful for who they are.

2. Questions to practice honoring yourself and your partner:

   - "Am I treating myself with regard and honoring what is true for me?"

   - "Am I treating my partner with regard and honoring their choices?"

3. Questions to practice trusting your own awareness:

   - "Am I trusting my own awareness?"

   - "Am I trusting my partner to do what they are going to do, regardless of what I think they should do?"

4. Questions to ask to have more vulnerability:

   - "Do I have barriers up right now?"

   - "Am I being vulnerable right now?"

5. Questions for expanding your allowance:

   - "Am I having allowance for myself?"

   - "Am I having allowance for my partner?"

   - "Does my allowance require expanding?"

6. Questions to practice using gratitude:

- "What am I grateful for about myself today?"

- "What am I grateful for about my partner today?"

Living The Five Elements of Intimacy with yourself and with your partner will ultimately create more harmony and ease, and enable you to have a deeper connection with one another.

Throughout the rest of this book, we will be exploring additional tools that will empower you to experience The Five Elements of Intimacy at a deeper level.

In the next chapter we will be guiding you on how to get out of making conclusions and into asking questions, so that you can start "Changing the Box of Relationship Into Living without Limits".

CHAPTER THREE

Getting Out of Conclusions and Into Asking Questions

~

"Would you rather be right or would you rather be free?"
Gary Douglas

I N THIS CHAPTER, we will begin to explore ways for getting you out of making conclusions and into asking questions for changing any area of your life. When you get out of the habit of making conclusions, and instead start functioning from your awareness, doors to new possibilities will begin to open.

Our conclusions come from a variety of different sources, such as our life experiences, our beliefs and other people's ideas that we have adopted as our own. We then believe these conclusions and fixed points of view about life to be fact and as a result no longer question them.

In the old paradigm, conclusions are an integral part of our cultural and social conditioning. On a personal level, our conclusions keep us locked into fixed points of view and end up limiting our choices. In a relationship, conclusions often create challenges, especially when we find ourselves defending what we believe to be right.

Have you ever known someone that fought for the rightness of their point of view as though no other choices were available? You may have also seen this on a global scale. How many wars and conflicts are based on conclusions and fixed points of view?

In the old paradigm, one of the major ways we create separation from our partners is when we hold onto the rightness of our points of view or the wrongness of our partner's points of view.

In the new paradigm, you are empowered to make choices. The tools we are presenting in this chapter are designed to empower you to make conscious choices.

'Good or Bad' or 'Right or Wrong'

Growing up, many people learned through conditioning and programming that they needed to get things right. Most of us have experienced parents or caregivers that taught us to place an enormous amount of significance on the rightness and the wrongness of our actions and choices.

Also, many people learned to withdraw their love when they concluded that the other person did something wrong. For many of us, we learned early on to avoid being made wrong, so that we could be right and earn the approval of others.

Our parents' conclusions about whether we were 'good or bad' or 'right or wrong' taught many of us to make conclusions about our own behavior, as well as the behavior of others. This often led us to functioning from within a "conclusionary reality". In other words, we functioned from our conclusions and fixed points of view rather than from our awareness and new possibilities.

Whenever we conclude that anything is 'good or bad' or 'right or wrong', it creates a limitation to receiving anything other than what we have already concluded. Let's say that you concluded: "That was the best sex I have ever had." While this statement may *seem* positive, it still limits being able to receive anything better than what you already decided was the best.

Alternatively, if you were to say, "Wow, that was amazing sex," *and* "What's it going to take for more of *that* to show up?", you allow yourself to continue to receive more. You can use this principle to create more receiving in any area of your life.

Likewise, if you concluded: "That was the worst service I have ever had," and therefore "I'm never going back to that restaurant!", you eliminate receiving anything other than what you have already concluded.

Alternatively, if you concluded: "That was really horrible service I had, " *and* "How does it get any better than this?", you continue to allow yourself to receive new possibilities. What if, by being open to new possibilities, you went back to the same restaurant the following week and had an amazing meal and service?

Interesting Point of View

"Your point of view creates your reality." Dr. Dain Heer

The way that most people see and interact with the world is through the filters of their conclusions and fixed points of view. From an early age we are taught that the world and our reality are what shape and create our points of view. This new model we are bringing forth empowers you to make choices 10 seconds at a time, and to be the creator of your own reality.

What if your point of view is what *actually* creates your reality? A similar concept is widely known in science as the "observer effect". This means that the act of observing something will influence that which is being observed. This means that when you notice something in your life that isn't working and you would like to change it, you can simply change your point of view about what isn't working, and this allows for a new possibility to show up.

Having an "interesting point of view", rather than a fixed point of view, means that you create freedom for yourself, regardless of other people's choices. For example, if your partner is in a bad mood, you can either have a fixed point of view that something is wrong, and that you also need to be in a bad mood or, alternatively, you can have an "interesting point of view" about the situation and therefore not be affected by it.

Playing with The Tool of Interesting Point of View

Your point of view creates your reality, so when you change your point of view, you change your reality. Here are examples of how you can use the tool of Interesting Point of View when you have a point of view that you would like to change.

If your partner is having an upset, and you find that you have the point of view that you need to be upset too, you can undo this point of view by saying either silently or out loud, three or more times: "Interesting point of view, I have this point of view. Interesting point of view, I have this point of view. Interesting point of view, I have this point of view." This will start to unravel your fixed point of view that has maintained the upset for you.

Another example: if you find yourself judging your body, you can start to undo this point of view by saying, "Interesting point of view, I have this point of view. Interesting point of view, I have this point of view. Interesting point of view, I have this point of view." This will start to unravel your fixed point of view that has maintained the judgment of your body.

Anytime you have an upset, you can also use this tool to remind yourself that your fixed points of view are just filters you have adopted and are not necessarily real, however real they may seem.

We will continue to explore using this tool as we move through the book.

Conclusions and Your Relationship

Conclusions have a profound impact on the way you relate to your partner. These include your general conclusions about life and also the fixed points of view you have about relationship. You may have been conditioned to believe that your partner should behave in a certain way. Many of our points of view about what we desire in relationship have been adopted from what is portrayed in love stories and love songs.

Growing up, many of us were taught to believe in 'the one and only true love', 'the knight in shining armor' or 'the prince on the white horse'. Much of the disappointment in relationship for many people comes from when the person they get into relationship with doesn't match the Hollywood version of what they have been entrained to desire.

Questions for getting out of conclusions and into new possibilities:

- "What else is possible?"

- "What questions can I ask to change this?"

- "What other choices are available?"

Asking and Receiving

The simplest way to get out of making conclusions is to ask questions. The basic premise of asking questions is that you are not attached to a fixed answer or an outcome. Attaching to a fixed outcome means that you've asked the question, but have already concluded what the answer should be.

If you try to control the outcome, it is likely that you will just be creating another conclusion about what the answer should be. In the new paradigm, asking questions is about being open to receiving awareness and new possibilities. It is also important to keep in mind that the awareness may not always come right away or in the form that you were expecting it to.

When you ask a question like "What other choices are available?", it will empower you to get out of conclusion and into the realm of possibility.

Ways of Formulating Questions

Throughout this book we will be empowering you to formulate questions. Below are examples of the differences between making a conclusion, making a conclusion with a question mark attached, and asking a question:

Conclusion: "I hate how fat my body is!"

Conclusion with a question mark attached: "What will it take to not have a fat body?"

Question: "What will it take to have more ease with my body?"

Notice in the first example that there is a conclusion that the body is fat. In the second example, there is still a conclusion that the body is fat—it just has a question mark attached on the end. In the third example, a real, open-ended question has been asked.

Here are other examples:

Conclusion: "You're a jerk for saying that!"

Conclusion with a question mark attached: "What will it take for you to not be a jerk?"

Question: "What did you intend by saying that?"

The basic premise here is that if you ask a question and you have already concluded what the answer should be, you won't receive anything other than what matches the answer that you have already decided upon.

What Will it Take to Change This?

Simply asking "What will it take to change this?" is a tool you can use for creating change in any area of your life. Asking this question starts to open up the door to new possibilities for you, even if you don't get the awareness of what that is, right away.

Here is an example of how to use this tool and to formulate additional questions with it:

- "What will it take to change my body?"

- "What will it take to change _____?"

- "What will it take to have more money?"

- "What will it take to have _____?"

We will be exploring this tool further in Chapter 8.

Destroying and Un-creating Your Limitations

As we highlighted in the acknowledgments of this book, most of the tools we are sharing with you have come from Access Consciousness, which was created by Gary Douglas. In Access Consciousness, there is a clearing statement which, when used in conjunction with asking a question, contributes to profound changes in any area of your life.

In this book, we are presenting a simplified version of this clearing statement. It involves asking a question for something you desire to change, and adding a statement that will "destroy and un-create" anything that doesn't allow it to change. (See *Resources* for the complete Access Consciousness clearing statement.)

In the simplified clearing statement, when you say you will "destroy and un-create" something that you desire to change, you are destroying and un-creating old, stuck energy that holds limitations in place, and this allows for new possibilities to arise. Destroying and un-creating is about getting rid of limitations and getting rid of the necessity of keeping those limitations as your only choice.

The following example shows how this works:

> A client came to us to facilitate a change for them. After they replied to a series of questions, it became evident that what was creating their limitation was the necessity of being 'a lone wolf '. When asked if they would destroy and un-create this limitation, they replied, "I like the idea of being a lone wolf." We explained that it wasn't destroying and un-creating the choice to be a lone wolf; rather, it was destroying and un-creating the limitation of the necessity for being a lone wolf as their one and only choice.

The following examples show how you can ask a question, and then follow it up by applying the simplified clearing statement for creating change:

- "What will it take for me to have more fun in my relationship?" *Anything that doesn't allow this, I will now destroy and un-create it all.*

- "What will it take for me to have more money?" *Anything that doesn't allow this, I will now destroy and un-create it all.*

- "What will it take to have more sex with my partner?" *Anything that doesn't allow this, I will now destroy and un-create it all.*

The simplified clearing statement will be used throughout the book in a variety of ways for creating change; sometimes you may need to say the same clearing multiple times.

Destroying and Un-creating Your Relationship Every Day

Using the tool of Destroying and Un-creating Your Relationship Every Day allows you to create your relationship anew every day *and* 10 seconds at a time. You are not *actually* destroying and un-creating the relationship. Rather, what you are destroying and un-creating are the limitations, expectations, projections, conclusions and judgments about the relationship.

How to apply this tool:

Every day, you can say: "Everything that my relationship was yesterday, I will now destroy and un-create it all."

NIRMADA: At the start of a relationship, people often function from conclusions about what the relationship should be, rather than asking questions and creating it 10 seconds at a time.

A reminder: The way to get out of making conclusions is to start asking questions, such as:

- "What else is possible?"

- "What other choices are available?"

- "What would be fun for us to create together today?"

Freedom Beyond the Limitations of Conclusions

In this chapter we started to explore ways for getting you out of making conclusions and into asking questions for changing any area of your life. When you stop looking for answers and start functioning from your awareness, you will begin to experience a new level of freedom in your life.

The tools throughout this book build upon themselves in a pragmatic way. We invite you to practice using them on a daily basis. When applied often, they have the possibility of changing and expanding every area of your life.

Tool Reminder: As previously mentioned, you can always ask for your allowance to expand when it's required. Remembering to expand your allowance is especially helpful, as your awareness *will* increase from using these tools.

Summary of the Tools, Concepts and Questions from Chapter Three

1. Conclusions and fixed points of view—These are the ways we have been entrained to see the world. We believe these conclusions and fixed points of view about life to be fact and as a result no longer question them.

2. The simplified clearing statement—"*Anything that doesn't allow this, I will now destroy and un-create it all.*" Apply this statement after asking a question for getting rid of limitations and creating a change.

3. "How does it get any better than this?"®—A question to ask when things are going well, and when things are not going well and you desire them to get better.

4. "What's it going to take for more of *that* to show up?"—A question to ask when you desire more of something to show up.

5. Questions to ask for getting out of conclusions and into new possibilities:

    *   "What else is possible?"

    *   "What questions can I ask to change this?"

    *   "What other choices are available?"

6. "Interesting point of view, I have this point of view." — A tool to get you out of a fixed point of view and into receiving new possibilities. We recommend that you say this three or more times.

In the next chapter, we will be exploring how you can begin to undo expectations and projections and continue to create a life and relationship you really desire.

CHAPTER FOUR

Living Beyond Expectations and Projections

~

IN THE NEW paradigm, we encourage you to practice getting out of the habit of using expectations and projections in your life and relationship. In this chapter, we are going to show you how using your awareness allows you to choose what works for you 10 seconds at a time.

In the old paradigm, as previously discussed, many people have a preconceived idea or conclusion about what their life and relationship should 'look like'. When we learn to let go of these expectations and projections of what we think our life and relationship should be, new unexpected possibilities begin to show up.

As this chapter unfolds, it will become more apparent how pervasive and normalized the use of expectations and projections has become. The tools presented in this chapter will begin to undo these limitations that you may have been imposing on your life and relationship. The more you practice using these tools in your daily life, the easier it will become.

The new paradigm invites you to consider the possibilities of:

- Being exactly as you are, without being controlled or affected by expectations and projections

- No longer trying to control the behavior of your partner, with the belief that you will be happier if they behave in ways you expect they should

- Having allowance for your partner to show up as they are

- Allowing your life and relationship to unfold 10 seconds at a time

If you have been attached to a fixed outcome in your relationship through expectations and projections, what would occur if you no longer had the need to control the outcome? When you are attached to a fixed outcome, this means you have already concluded what you can or can't receive.

When you live beyond expectations and projections, and you regularly ask the question "What else is possible?", you open yourself up to new possibilities and choices you never knew existed.

Expectations and Projections in The Old Paradigm

In the old paradigm, from the moment we arrive on Earth, we are expected throughout our lives to act and behave in certain ways. Many of the expectations and projections in relationship have come from the perpetuation of love stories and love songs that are prevalent in our culture.

When we meet someone for the first time, and there is a connection or chemistry, many people begin projecting right away about how it would be if they were with this other person. These projected futures are often made before we even get to know the other person. Some people even go so far as to picture their wedding day and growing old together.

In the old paradigm, when we start projecting onto our partner and relationship, it creates a 'design blueprint', and then this 'blueprint' gets locked into place. The relationship then has limited possibilities to evolve and grow beyond what we have already projected it should be.

How many of us have ever concluded, "This is the perfect man (or woman) for me!" If we make a conclusion like this and then our partner becomes critical or judgmental, for example, we can find ourselves still locked into the initial conclusion that they are the perfect person for us.

As previously highlighted, when we conclude that something is a certain way, we then cut off our awareness to anything other than what we have already concluded. If we had concluded that we would be with someone forever, even if it wasn't working for us anymore, we would have already cut off our awareness to having the ease of knowing that other choices were available.

A New Paradigm of Relationship — Beyond Expectations and Projections

In the new paradigm, you learn to be aware of what works for you and know that you have a new choice available in every 10 seconds. When things aren't working for you, you know you can ask, "What other choices are available?"

In contrast to being locked into staying with someone forever as your only choice, in this new model, you have the willingness to lose the other person and this gives you the freedom of choice. Ironically, the willingness to lose the other person can actually allow you to change the box of relationship into living together without limits.

As you let go of your expectations and projections, you can then choose to be with your partner, 10 seconds at a time, without concluding that anything in the relationship needs to be locked into place.

A reminder: The willingness to lose someone doesn't mean you actually *have* to lose them. It means that you have the freedom to choose what works for you, 10 seconds at a time. This ultimately creates more intimacy, harmony and ease with you and your partner.

The Old Paradigm vs. The New Paradigm

The following chart contains some sample statements showing the difference between functioning from the old paradigm and functioning in the new paradigm.

Old Paradigm	New Paradigm
You need to change.	I could expand my allowance right now.
How could you have done that?	That's an interesting choice.
You hurt my feelings.	Interesting point of view, I have this point of view.
That doesn't work.	What else is possible?
You must do it this way.	What other choices are available?

Destroying and Un-creating your Expectations and Projections

One of the easiest ways to move beyond expectations and projections is to destroy and un-create all the expectations and projections that you have put on your relationship, yourself and your partner every day.

This allows you to create your life and relationship, 10 seconds at time, beyond the expectations and projections that keep you from living without limits. By doing so, you will be on the creative edge of creating your life and relationship every day, rather than concluding them out of possibility.

A reminder: Destroying and un-creating expectations and projections is done in order to clear old, stuck energy that holds limitations in place. This allows for new possibilities to arise.

How do you move beyond expectations and projections? Simply say every day:

- "All the expectations and projections I have about my relationship, I will now destroy and un-create them all."

- "All the expectations and projections I have about myself, I will now destroy and un-create them all."

- "All the expectations and projections I have about my partner, I will now destroy and un-create them all."

- "All the expectations and projections that others have about me, I will now destroy and un-create them all."

When you begin living beyond expectations and projections, an entirely new world of possibility and choice will open up for your life and relationship.

Choice Creates Awareness

When you move beyond functioning from expectations and projections, you use your awareness for choosing what works for you, 10 seconds at a time. Every choice creates something, as choice is the source of creation.

The following tools will show you how you can make choices that work for you so that you can begin to perceive the energy of what those choices will create. We invite you to practice using these tools on a daily basis.

Perceiving Your Light and Heavy for Making Choices

Perceiving Your Light and Heavy is a tool you can apply to knowing what's true for you (what works for you) and what's not true for you (what doesn't work for you). There is no right or wrong way to perceive what's "light" and "heavy" for *you* as it is different for each person. We invite you to practice using this tool so you become familiar with perceiving *your* "light" and *your* "heavy".

Perceiving the energy of your light or heavy is about becoming aware of your body's sensations. Most people call these sensations 'feelings'; and what we are referring to here is learning to perceive the awareness that your body is giving you.

Using the tool of Perceiving Your Light and Heavy is a way of making choices from a place of expansion and possibility, rather than from one of contraction and conclusion. We've talked a lot in this book about making choices in 10-second increments and being clear as to what does and doesn't work for you. Once you establish what your light is and what your heavy is, you can use this awareness to make choices that work for you.

A reminder: What is light and works for you in one 10 seconds may not be light or work for you in the next 10 seconds.

Some of the ways you might perceive *your* light are: a weight has been lifted; you are more expansive, super excited, breathing easier, joyful and happy; you have a surge of enthusiasm, tingles, and you are uplifted. Remember, there is no right or wrong here, as your light is your own unique way of perceiving energy.

Some of the ways you might perceive *your* heavy are: you are weighed down, contracted, melancholy, disinterested, unhappy, dull, suppressed; you know that something just isn't right. Remember, there is no right or wrong here as your heavy is your own unique way of perceiving energy.

Here are some examples of how you can start to practice Perceiving Your Light and Heavy. If someone yelled "You're ugly!" at you, would that make you feel light or heavy? It most likely makes you feel heavy, as you know it's not true. If someone said "You're an amazing person," to you, does that make you feel light or heavy? It most likely makes you feel light and expansive.

For instance, if someone named Sally were taking a lie detector test, most likely she would be asked, "Is your name Sally?" If she replied "Yes", this would create a lightness and expansion in her body as this is true. And if she replied "No", this would create a heaviness and contraction in her body, as this is not true. The lie detector test would pick up what's true and not true in a very similar way to how you perceive what's light and heavy for you.

We invite you to ask questions daily and practice using the tool of Perceiving Your Light and Heavy to learn how to make choices that work for you. One way to start to perceive the energy of your light is to say a statement that you know is true and then perceive the sensations in your body. Also, to practice perceiving the energy of your heavy, you can say a statement that you know is not true and then perceive the sensations in your body.

For example, if it's Monday and you say, "It's Monday," then this is true and notice what you perceive. If it's Monday and you say, "It's Wednesday," then this is not true. Notice what you perceive. You can continue practicing the tool of Perceiving Your Light and Heavy by applying it to anything you know is true or not true.

A reminder: The tool of Expanding Your Allowance is very useful when you practice learning to perceive energy. Many people don't perceive energy right away, so we invite you to have allowance for yourself as you practice something new. Additionally, as you become more aware from using these tools, expanding your allowance will create more ease.

If I Choose This, What Will My Life Be Like in Five Years?

Another tool you can use for moving beyond expectations and projections and into choice and possibility, is asking the question, "If I choose this what will my life be like in five years?"

This question is a practical tool for making choices about anything in your life and relationship, without going into conclusion about what the outcome will be. When you ask this question, it's not to conclude what your life would be like in five years; rather, you ask it so you can perceive the energy of what your choice will create.

For example, if you concluded you wanted to buy a particular car, you could ask, "If I choose to buy this car, what will my life be like in five years?" After asking this, if you perceive the energy as heavy, it is a clear indication that that's a choice that doesn't work for you.

Alternatively, if you were to ask, "If I don't choose to buy this car, what will my life be like in five years?" and you perceive the energy as light, this would be a clear indication that your choice to *not* buy the car was going to work for you.

Another example is: if your partner asked you if you would like to go to a party, you could ask, "If I choose to go to this party, what will my life be like in five years?" After asking this, if you perceive the energy as light, this would be a clear indication that your choice to go to the party was going to work for you.

JOHN: As highlighted in our personal story, when I first met Nirmada, I was in a mining job that no longer worked for me, but I had concluded I needed to stay in the job as though it was my only choice. There was a perpetual conflict going on, as I could perceive the heaviness that this job was no longer working for me and yet, I had also concluded that I needed the money so I couldn't leave.

One day, I was having a really rough day at work, and that's when I made the demand that something had to change. I asked, "If I leave this job, what will my life be like in five years?" I immediately perceived a surge of light and expansive energy and I knew that by leaving this job, it was going to create something far greater for me. I didn't at the time know what that 'far greater' was; however the energy I perceived was so energetically light that I knew the choice of leaving the job was going to work for me. This choice to leave, though not cognitive, opened up a whole new set of possibilities that has expanded every area of my life.

Making choices in 10-second increments and following the energy of perceiving what's light or heavy for you is not about getting it 'right or wrong' or 'good or bad'. It's really about learning to follow the energy of what you desire to invite into your life and what works for you.

For example, if you desire to create an expansive and joyful life, and you follow your awareness of what's light and works for you, then you are inviting expansive and joyful things into your life.

Summary of the Tools, Concepts and Questions from Chapter Four

1. Expectations and projections — In the old paradigm, the preconceived ideas or conclusions about what our life or relationship should 'look like'.

2. Destroying and un-creating — Every day, you destroy and un-create all the expectations and projections that you have of your relationship, yourself and your partner. This is one of the easiest ways to create your life and relationship, 10 seconds at time.

3. Perceiving Your Light and Heavy for making choices — A tool you can apply for knowing what's true

for you (what works for you) and what's not true for you (what doesn't work for you).

4. "If I choose this, what will my life be like in five years?" — A practical tool for making choices about anything in your life and relationship without getting into a conclusion about what the outcome will be.

Love in the Next 10 Seconds has introduced you to many new tools and core concepts for creating your new paradigm in relationship. In the next part of the book we'll be exploring some new tools, and how to put them into practice in your everyday life, alongside Making Choices in 10-Second Increments.

PART TWO

Practicing the Tools For a New Kind of Relationship

CHAPTER FIVE

"Who Does This Belong To?" and "Is This Really Mine?"

~

IN THE NEW paradigm, when you begin functioning from your awareness, rather than from cultural and social conditioning, you start to realize that not *all* of your thoughts, feelings and emotions are your own. The normalized reality of thoughts, feelings and emotions based on trauma and drama from the old paradigm will begin to become a thing of the past. In the new paradigm, we show you how to access your awareness for creating a life and relationship you really desire.

When we first suggest to people that not *all* of their thoughts, feelings and emotions belong to them, it can push their buttons. You may be experiencing something similar to this right now. In this book we are sharing tools and questions that are designed to clear out old patterns and stuck energy that don't actually belong to you, and this allows for new freedom and new possibilities to arise.

Have you ever had a melancholy feeling for no apparent reason? Have you ever become unexpectedly happy or furious and had no idea why? Our question to you is: What if you're just more psychic and aware than you have ever acknowledged?

In the old paradigm, most of us have been taught to believe that *all* of our thoughts, feelings and emotions *must* belong to us, rather than recognizing how perceptive we actually are. Have you ever felt like you were living someone else's life or that you weren't being yourself and you just didn't know why? The following tools will allow you to be empowered to know what's yours and what doesn't actually belong to you.

Using the Tool of "Who Does This Belong To?"

Asking silently or out loud, "Who does this belong to?" is an effective tool to use when you find you're not being like yourself, are feeling stuck, or just know that something needs to change. After asking "Who does this belong to?" about any thoughts, feelings, or emotions you have that seem heavy and not true for you, the heavy feeling will dissipate or become lighter if the thoughts, feelings and emotions don't *actually* belong to you.

As previously mentioned, when you perceive something as light, it's true for you, and when you perceive something as heavy, it's not true for you. The tools of Light and Heavy and "Who Does This Belong To?" go hand in hand.

Let's say that you are driving down the street and all of a sudden you become angry for no reason. In the old paradigm you might just assume that the anger is yours, not question it and continue to be angry. In the new paradigm, in this same situation, you might ask, "Who does *that* belong to?" and if the angry feeling goes away or dissipates, you'll know that it doesn't belong to you.

After you have the awareness that the anger doesn't belong to you, you might even, for instance, look at the car next to you and notice that the person driving the car is yelling angrily at the passenger. People are very much like satellite dishes and radio receivers, picking up and perceiving the energies of everyone and everything around them.

When you ask, "Who does this belong to?", it's a way of letting go of anything you are perceiving that is not *actually* yours. It's not relevant where the thoughts, feelings and emotions came from: what's important is that you are *now* allowing yourself to let go of holding onto things that are *not* actually yours.

In the new paradigm, practicing these tools will allow you to begin acknowledging your awareness, rather than assuming everything you are aware of must belong to you. Have you ever gone onto something like Facebook and then suddenly found yourself in an annoyed mood for no reason? Was that really *your* annoyed mood or was it your *awareness* of the millions of people on the World Wide Web that were in an annoyed mood?

Here are some examples from everyday life that show how aware people really are and how this often goes unacknowledged. For instance, when somebody hugs you and it's super warm and fuzzy, have you ever perceived this energy? If yes, this is you perceiving what you are aware of. If somebody hugs you and it's cold and rigid, have you ever perceived this energy? If yes, this is also you perceiving what you are aware of. Have you ever thought about someone and then they instantaneously call you?

What if you are far more aware than you have ever given yourself credit for? Many people have been conditioned into not acknowledging their awareness; we encourage you to practice using these tools daily.

The tool of "Who Does This Belong To?" has been used for over 15 years with amazing results from all over the World. Many years ago, Dr. Dain Heer, chiropractor and co-creator of Access Consciousness, had a patient with back pain that he treated for three months without success. Finally, Dain asked the patient, "Since nothing else has worked, I am going to ask you a really weird question, and just give me the first thing that comes into your head. Who does this pain belong to?" The patient blurted out, "My wife!" Dain said, "Did your wife ever have anything like this?" He said, "Yes, several years ago she had bad back pain and I remember thinking I would do anything to get her out of pain. Three months later, I developed back pain in the exact same place." Dain asked, " How's your back now?" The patient said, "Oh my goodness, it's 70% better!"

Dain was amazed that asking "Who does this belong to?" changed the patient's back pain instantaneously when no other technique had worked. Dain then discovered in his chiropractic practice that somewhere between 50% and 90% of the pain in people's bodies could be eliminated by asking them "Who does this belong to?" or "Is this really yours?"

Using the Tool of "Is This Really Mine?"

Asking silently or out loud "Is this really mine?" is another effective tool to use when you find you are not acting like yourself, are feeling heavy, or just know you desire something to change. After asking "Is this really mine?" for any thoughts, feelings, or emotions you have that seem heavy and not true for you, if the thoughts, feelings and emotions don't actually belong to you, the heavy feeling will dissipate and become lighter.

JOHN: One afternoon, I had a really intense headache. Nirmada asked, "Is that headache really yours?" The moment she asked this question, the intensity of my headache dissipated. Once I got the awareness that the headache wasn't actually mine, this allowed for it to change.

NIRMADA: One day, I was having some challenges. John asked, "What's going on?" and I yelled back, "I'm in a really bad mood." He replied, "Can I ask you a question? Is that bad mood really yours?" I chuckled and immediately knew that it wasn't, and instantly I felt better and lighter. When I believed the bad mood was mine, everything was heavy for me. When I realized that none of it was mine, everything shifted.

The Origin of "Who Does This Belong To?"

Gary Douglas had always struggled with the non-stop thoughts in his head. One day, many years ago, he was meditating and noticed his thoughts were about him needing to do the laundry, except he never did laundry: his wife did. Also, thoughts about needing to clean the windows came up and this was something he never did. He asked, "Are any of these thoughts mine?" and got a 'no'. He started asking, "Who does this belong to?" for every thought, feeling and emotion he had, and every thought, feeling and emotion that wasn't his would dissipate or go away. He realized he was perceiving a constant inflow of other people's thoughts, feelings and emotions, and that they didn't actually belong to him.

Once you practice using the tool of "Who Does This Belong To?", you will still be aware of other people's thoughts, feelings, and emotions; however, you'll be able to let go of the burden of being affected by things that aren't actually yours.

Playing with Using "Who Does This Belong to?" and "Is This Really Mine?"

First and foremost, what would it take for you to have fun playing with using these tools? For instance, the next time you suddenly get upset, angry or irritated, you can simply ask "Who does *this* belong to?" or "Is this *really* mine?"

There is no right or wrong way of using these tools. If something isn't yours, it will dissipate and go away after asking these questions. Sometimes, you might even start to smile and laugh as things lighten up for you.

A reminder: This is not cognitive or logical, and the worst thing that can occur when you use these tools is that you will let go of the burden of being affected by things that aren't actually yours.

Imagine a landfill with all the trash from a major city. Can you perceive the heavy energy of this landfill if you were sitting in the middle of it? Now, imagine a warm tropical beach at sunset. Can you perceive the lightness and the joyful energy of sitting on this beach? When we buy the 'crap' of the old paradigm, it's like sitting in the middle of a landfill. When you apply the tools of "Who Does This Belong To?" and "Is This Really Mine?", you will gain the awareness that the 'crap' of this reality isn't actually yours, and this will give you the choice of "sitting on the beach at sunset".

When someone watches the news and a horrible event takes place, they often feel horrible while watching it and possibly for a long time afterwards. If someone watches TV with an amazing story, they often feel uplifted, both during and afterwards. Have you ever been in a great mood, and then had a family member call who was having a horrible day and after the call, you felt horrible too?

So, what if, by acknowledging how aware you are and by practicing the tools in this book, every mood you have could just be a choice, 10 seconds at a time?

If It's Not Mine, then Whose Is It?

What's important is knowing that not *every* thought, feeling, and emotion you are aware of is yours, and that you now have tools to let go of the burden of holding onto them. It's not relevant where the thoughts, feelings or emotions originated from. For instance, if you were in a crowded room and someone broke wind, would you rather leave the situation behind, or stay, smell the odor and find out where it came from?

In this book we have been sharing tools and concepts for creating freedom in every area of your life. This is about empowering you to know that your awareness, through asking questions, is more powerful than anyone else's answer.

How many times in your life have you been told to do something a certain way because someone else told you that that's the way it's done? An example of this comes from a story, where a new bride is making her first dinner for her husband. She's making her mother's brisket recipe, cutting off the ends of the roast. Her husband asks, "Why are you cutting off the ends — that's the best part!" She replies, "That's the way my mother always made it." The bride asks her mother, "Why do you cut off the ends of the roast?" Her mother replies, "That's the way my mother always made it." The bride then asks her grandmother, "Why do you cut off the ends of the roast?" Her grandmother replies, "That's the only way it fits in my pan."

In the old paradigm, how many of us have been told erroneous things throughout our lives, spoken as though they were true, and based on someone else's conclusion? Another example of this is the 'telephone game'. It's played around the world — one person whispers a message into the ear of another, who then whispers it to another, who then whispers it to another...

until the last player announces the message to the entire group. Errors typically accumulate in the retellings, so the statement announced by the last player differs significantly from the original message.

How many times do people eat something and afterwards say, "Why did I eat that? I wasn't even hungry!" People often assume that the thoughts in their head to eat something are actually their own, rather than asking a question like "Is this hunger *really* mine or just my awareness of someone else's body?" Oftentimes, after asking this question, if the hunger is not actually yours, the desire to eat will go away.

So, it's not actually relevant where all your thoughts, feelings, and emotions originated from; what is important to remember is that they are not all yours. The good news is that you now have tools to use daily for knowing what's true for you and making choices that work for you, 10 seconds at a time.

Asking "Who Does This Belong To?" for Three Days

A tremendous freedom can be created by asking for three days, "Who does this belong to?" for every thought, feeling, and emotion you have. Three consecutive days of asking "Who does this belong to?" has the possibility of breaking you free from the non-stop cycle of believing that every thought, feeling and emotion you are perceiving is actually yours.

A reminder: When you ask "Who does this belong to?" or "Is this really mine?" for every thought, feeling and emotion you have, if you feel lighter after asking these questions, then the thoughts, feelings, and emotions were not yours, and will naturally dissipate.

JOHN: Some years ago, after choosing to ask "Who does this belong to?" for three consecutive days, many changes occurred. On the first day, I consistently asked this question and didn't notice much change. On the second day, I had to ask this question many times and started to notice that some things were changing, though I couldn't have said exactly what they were.

On the afternoon of the third day, just as I was wondering if this tool actually worked, a wave of peace suddenly came over me. Everything around me became quiet and still even though I was driving a vehicle on a gravel road. It was like all the background noise of other people's thoughts, feelings and emotions had turned off inside my head. I was in a state of a 'walking meditation' and knew at this moment that using this tool consistently for three days really does work.

NIRMADA: Asking "Who does this belong to?" consistently for three days opened up my life to a whole new world of possibilities. During the time I did this exercise, I lived by myself, on a nature reserve in total privacy. I chose to stay inside for the entire three days, without communicating with the outside world. That included turning off the computer and phone. The number of times that I was required to ask "Who does this belong to?" for every thought, feeling and emotion that went through my head was astounding to me as I was not having any physical communication with the outside world.

This three-day exercise allowed me to acknowledge how aware and psychic I really am and set me free me from believing that all of the thoughts, feelings and emotions I am aware of are mine. For example, I had always assumed I was really bad at relationship. After I met John, I realized I am really good at relationship. Once I started applying the tool of "Who Does This Belong To?", I realized that none of my previous thoughts, feelings or emotions about relationship were even mine in the first place.

What About the Good Thoughts?

The challenge for some people with using the tool of "Who Does This Belong To?" is that they realize that even some of the good thoughts don't actually belong to them.

One example of freeing yourself from believing that the good thoughts must also all belong to you comes from one of our clients. One day, she was flirting with a contact on Facebook and became aware of warm and fuzzy, turned-on feelings. She remembered the tools of "Who Does This Belong To?" and "Is This Really Mine?" and she put them to the test. When she asked, "Is this warm and fuzzy, turned-on feeling really mine?" she got a 'no' and realized that it was her awareness of the other person's turn-on.

She realized that if she had bought that the warm and fuzzy, turned-on feelings were her own, when they weren't, this would have cut off her awareness and limited her choices. It became much lighter and easier for her to acknowledge that it was the other person's point of view. This enabled her to see what was true for her by asking, "What's *my* point of view here?" The awareness she got from asking this question was: it was fun for her to flirt and to have this person lust after her body. This ultimately created more fun, freedom and choice for her.

Is This Judgment Really Mine?

How often do we have a judgmental thought about someone that we have never spoken to and don't even know? What if these judgmental thoughts don't actually belong to us? Oftentimes, we are just aware of the other person's judgment of themselves or their judgment of others. Practicing using "Who does this belong to?" and "Is this really mine?" is an easy way to start living beyond judgment.

NIRMADA: One day at the gym, I started having judgments about my body. I asked, "Are any of these judgments mine?" After I asked this question, the thoughts lightened up and went away. I realized that none of the judgments were mine and that they were actually my awareness of the judgments that others had about their own bodies.

"Who Am I Being Right Now?"

When you find that you are not acting like yourself, you can ask, "Who am I being right now?" or "Am I being me?" When you ask these questions, you can become aware of when you are not being yourself or when you have bought other people's thoughts, feelings and emotions as your own. A classic example of how this works for many people, once they start asking questions like this, is when they start talking like one of their parents and then say things like, "I just sounded exactly like my mother."

Sometimes, when required and done in a kind and contributing way, you can also ask your partner, "Who are you being right now?" or "Are you being you?" Asking these questions can often pull someone out of believing that every thought, feeling and emotion is their own.

Is This Really Ours?

As well as asking if something belongs to you, you can ask a similar question when there are challenges in relationship.

Just as you can perceive the thoughts, feelings and emotions of others and buy into them as your own, you may also find yourself doing the same in relationship. When you or your partner start acting in ways that don't seem true to who you are collectively in relationship, you can ask, "Are we being us right now?" If the energy gets lighter and dissipates after asking this question, it is an indicator that none of it was yours in the first place.

JOHN: Nirmada and I were out driving in a car one day. We suddenly found ourselves for no reason bickering and defending our points of view. When we asked, "Are we being us right now?", we got a 'no' and realized that we were just aware of the couple arguing at the house we had just been visiting. Everything became lighter and dissipated once we asked this question and then became aware that none of the thoughts, feelings and emotions that instigated the bickering were ours.

NIRMADA: We've interviewed many different couples from around the world that are choosing to create a new paradigm in relationship. One of the things we've discovered with almost every couple is that whenever they argue or fight, they now realize they are not being themselves and that nothing they argue about actually belongs to either of them.

What's So Right About Me That I'm Not Getting?

Love in The Next 10 Seconds has been created for empowering you to know that you are an amazing person, who can be and do anything you really desire. The tools are designed for you to become more aware, and to know that the 'crap' of the old paradigm is just not yours.

Using these tools will allow you to begin creating a life and relationship that works for you. Any time you require a little inspiration for the greatness of you, or if you are feeling a little heavy, you can always ask, "What's so right about me that I'm not getting?" Asking this question will begin to open up the door for your living without limits.

Summary of the Tools, Concepts and Questions from Chapter Five

1. "Who Does This Belong To? and "Is This Really Mine?" —Questions to ask when you feel like you are not being yourself or you are believing that *all* of your thoughts, feelings and emotions are your own.

2. "Who am I being right now?" and "Am I being me?' — Questions you can ask when you realize you are not being like yourself.

3. " Is this judgment really mine?" — A question to ask when you are believing that the judgments you are aware of are your own.

4. "Are we being us right now?" — A question to ask when something is occurring in your relationship that doesn't seem to belong to you or your partner.

5. "What's so right about me that I'm not getting?" — A question you can ask any time you are not being empowered to recognize the amazing person you really are.

Now that you are becoming more aware of the difference between what belongs to you and what doesn't belong to you, in the next chapter we'll be exploring how to begin creating your life and relationship beyond judgment.

CHAPTER SIX

Creating Relationship Beyond Judgment

~

"Consciousness includes everything and judges nothing."
Gary Douglas

IN THE NEW paradigm, you are encouraged to make choices in 10-second increments, and also to have allowance for the choices that your partner makes in 10-second increments. This allows you to function from your awareness and beyond the limitations of judgment.

When you start functioning from your awareness, rather than judgment, doors to new possibilities begin to open. In this chapter, we will explore tools for getting you out of judgment and into asking questions for enjoying every area of your life and relationship.

What is Judgment Really?

Judgment is an integral part of the way we function in the old paradigm. We are often taught to judge everything as 'right or wrong' or 'good or bad', rather than being curious and asking questions. Asking questions is an easy way to get out of judgment and into making choices 10 seconds at a time.

As previously highlighted, whenever we judge anything as 'right or wrong' or 'good or bad', it creates a limitation in receiving anything beyond what we have already concluded is possible.

For instance, if you meet someone and judge, "They're the *best* lover I ever had and I'm sure they're my soul mate!", and they stop being a great lover or partner for you, you may find it challenging to see anything beyond what you have already concluded they are to you. The well-known expression 'wearing rose-colored glasses' is an example of how this 'filtering system' works.

Alternatively, if you choose to not look through rose-colored glasses, you will allow yourself to see things as they are. For instance, if you meet someone and they are a great lover, you might ask, "What's it going to take for more of *that* to show up?"

By asking this question, the possibility of having more fun with this person can show up again, without cutting off your awareness. And, it might be just as good or *better* than it was before. Or, it might not actually work for you anymore. Either way, it's about not cutting off your awareness by judging what's 'right or wrong' or 'good or bad', and it is about making choices that work for you, 10 seconds at a time.

Is This a Judgment or an Awareness?

Judgment is always a choice and a primary source for creating limitation. Judgments can be negative points of view, and they can also be positive points of view. Oftentimes, people confuse a judgment as an awareness and an awareness as a judgment. An awareness can be of something that is considered either negative or positive.

If you have an awareness of something that is considered negative, it doesn't necessarily make it a judgment. For instance, if you are aware that someone is being unkind, and you say, "That was unkind," it isn't necessarily a judgment. However, if you then have a fixed point of view about the unkindness and you have labeled it as right or wrong, then you have moved into judgment.

Anytime you categorize what you're aware of as 'good or bad' or 'right or wrong', it becomes a judgment. Judgments always create limitations, whether they're negative or positive. Judgments solidify things into place and this then doesn't allow for the possibility for things to change.

There is a distinct difference between an awareness and a judgment. For clarity, you can ask, "Is this a judgment or an awareness?" Many people judge themselves for being judgmental when they are actually just being observant and aware.

Positive judgments, though they may seem positive, can still create limitations and are different from awareness. Let's look at how this works.

If someone says, "I like my body," this is actually a positive judgment. How often do you hear someone say, "I enjoy my body"? Liking something is a judgment based on 'good or bad' or 'right or wrong'. Enjoying your body is about having joy and pleasure with your body and is different from liking it, as it requires no judgment.

Whenever we use negative or positive judgments, it doesn't allow for anything greater to show up than what we've already judged. If you were to positively judge, "I have the best relationship," this judgment, though positive, may not allow for any greater possibility to show up with your relationship. Alternatively, you could say, "I have a great relationship," and "How does it get better than this?"

If you were to say, "I have the worst relationship!", you are not in allowance for any new possibilities to show up. Alternatively, you could say, " My relationship isn't working for me," and "What else is possible?"

Asking "How does it get better than this?" or "What else is possible?" opens the door to new possibilities in every situation of your life and relationship and begins the adventure of living without limits.

Is This Judgment Really Mine?

As we mentioned before, when you begin functioning from your awareness, rather than from cultural and social conditioning, you start to realize that not *all* of your judgments are your own.

The previously discussed tool of "Who Does This Belong To?" can be applied to judgment. In the old paradigm, we are taught that all of our thoughts, feelings and emotions are significant and that they all *must* belong to us. In the new paradigm, you realize that you are very aware of other people's thoughts, feelings and emotions and that they don't *all* belong to you.

A reminder: What's light for you is true and what's heavy for you isn't true. If you find yourself heavy and in judgment, you can ask these questions:

- "Is this judgment really mine?"

- "Who does this judgment belong to?"

After asking these questions, if the heaviness lightens up or goes away, then you know that the judgment wasn't yours. Also, when someone judges you, does that feel light or heavy to you? Most likely it feels heavy to you, as judgment is a creation and isn't real or true.

Judgment and Money

Money is a topic which invites many judgments in the old paradigm. How many judgments around money did we learn as children? Here are just a few: money is dirty; money doesn't grow on trees; you can't afford that; it's too expensive; rich people are unhappy; if I have money, people will try to steal it, and so on.

If you were to say "I never have enough money!", can you perceive the heaviness and limitation that's created from this judgment?

Alternatively, what if you desired more money and asked, "What's it going to take to have more money?" Can you perceive the lightness and possibility that is created by asking this question?

Questions and statements to create more possibilities with money:

- "What other choices are available about money that I have never considered before?"

- "What else is possible with money that I have never considered before?"

- "Is this really my point of view about money?"

- "All the limitations I have with money, I will now destroy and un-create them all."

- "Money come, money come, money come!"

Love and Judgment

Love in the Next 10 Seconds was written for creating freedom and possibility with loving and living in 10-second increments.

A reminder: What works for you in one 10 seconds may not work for you in the next 10 seconds. When you're making choices based on what's light and expansive for you, in 10-second increments, it's a way of having and creating love beyond judgment.

In the old paradigm, let's say a person meets someone new and judges, "I love you so much and you are the perfect person for me!" They might continue on to judge, "I have total unconditional love for you and I know that you will love me unconditionally forever!"

Unconditional love means something different to every person. Have you ever considered how many judgments are used to create the thing we call unconditional love? As time passes and one or both partners start to do things that upset or irritate the other, how quickly does the unconditional love turn into conditional love?

For instance, when someone says, "I love you unconditionally," what do they mean? Do they love you unconditionally when you anger them, or do they judge you for doing something wrong?

Alternatively, if you're just grateful for someone, then you can be grateful for them even when they anger you. Gratitude and judgment cannot exist at the same time. When you are grateful for someone, there is no separation or judgment and this allows for the gratitude to grow.

One traditional wedding vow is: "I'll love you until death do us part." Can you perceive the energy of this? Is it light and expansive or heavy and contracted? We recently attended a wedding in New Zealand and some of the light and expansive wedding vows were: "I'll love you 10 seconds at a time," "I'll be grateful for you," and "I'll have allowance for you."

Beyond Judgment and into Receiving

Judgment is an integral part of the way we function in the old paradigm of relationship and is used as a way of not receiving from our partners. Many people are taught to have fixed points of view about who they think their partner should be, and then judge them if they don't conform or live up to those expectations.

Whenever we judge our partner as being either 'right or wrong' or 'good or bad', this cuts off our receiving and awareness. For example, if you were having a conversation with your partner, and you became aware that they were not receiving what you were saying, you might make yourself wrong. Or, you might attempt to make them wrong for not receiving what you were saying.

Alternatively, if you are speaking with your partner and you become aware that they're not receiving what you're saying, rather than judging this as 'good or bad' or 'right or wrong', you could perceive it as just an awareness. Trusting your awareness, without having to judge what you're aware of, creates a freedom and ease for *you*, regardless of your partner's choices.

A reminder: Receiving is about receiving awareness. Therefore, if you practice not judging what's right or wrong about the things that you're aware of, the door opens to the possibilities of living without limits.

In the new paradigm, when we learn to have allowance for our own choices as well as our partner's choices, we stop cutting off parts and pieces of ourselves to maintain the relationship. This level of freedom allows us to get out of judgment and into receiving.

One of the ways people in relationship cut off receiving and cut off parts and pieces of themselves is when their partner judges that it's wrong to look at or admire someone else's body. People often don't consider how much enjoyment the body receives from looking at other people's bodies.

What if one partner in the relationship could receive from the other partner when they're looking at other people's bodies? What if this allowed your body and your partner's body to be more turned on than ever before and contributed to expanding your intimacy together?

Have you ever tried holding onto water? If you try to hold onto water by grasping it tightly in your fist, you will not be able to hold the water. However, if you cup your hands together gently, you will be able to embrace the water and it will remain naturally in your hands.

This metaphor applies to relationship. When you try to hold onto your partner through judging what they can and can't do, it's like trying to hold water in a tight fist. However, when you allow your partner to be who they are naturally without judging them, it's similar to embracing and receiving the water in your cupped hands.

Receiving beyond judgment includes knowing what does and doesn't work for you and using your awareness to make these choices. This is really what *Love in the Next 10 Seconds* is all about.

The Enjoyment of Sex Beyond Judgment

Many people have learned to have sex in judgment and not in the enjoyment of it. When judgment is present in lovemaking and sex, our capacity to receive our partner and to be received by our partner is limited.

What if we could receive everything in lovemaking, and not have the point of view that something needs to be judged as 'right or wrong' or 'good or bad'? If there were no significance attached to the outcome of lovemaking, how much more could we actually receive? What if sex and lovemaking could be a kind, caring and nurturing enjoyment of bodies beyond any of the judgments from the old paradigm?

Being seen through the eyes of someone that has no judgment of you or your body can be an expansive and orgasmic experience. As an example, many of us as young children freely ran around naked in front of other people without having any judgment that it was right or wrong. What would it be like to see yourself through the eyes of no judgment?

All the tools throughout this book are designed to get you out of judgment and into question, choice and possibility. So what questions can you ask that will open up your choices to new possibilities with the enjoyment of sex beyond judgment?

Questions and clearings for the enjoyment of sex:

- "What am I grateful for about my body?"

- "What am I grateful for about my partner's body?"

- "What else is possible with the enjoyment of sex?"

- "What's it going to take to have more enjoyment with sex?"

- "What other choices are available with the enjoyment of sex?"

- "All the judgments I have about sex, I will now destroy and un-create them all."

- "Anything that doesn't allow me to have the enjoyment of sex, I will now destroy and un-create it all."

Interesting Point of View and Judgment

Judgment is a choice and a creation, so anytime we are in judgment, it's created from a point of view of, or belief in, something we have decided is either 'right or wrong' or 'good or bad'. There's little freedom in our life and relationship when we have fixed points of view. Whenever we align and agree with, or resist and react to anyone or anything, this requires us to judge the rightness or wrongness of our points of view.

When you get out of having a 'fixed point of view' and into having an "interesting point of view", you are having allowance for what you previously judged as flaws, quirks, or faults about your partner.

As previously highlighted, your point of view creates your reality. So when you are having a point of view that's creating a judgment or separation, and you change your point of view, you'll be able to create beyond separation and judgment.

Tool Reminder: Interesting Point of View

The next time you find yourself in judgment you can say:

- "Interesting point of view, I have this point of view. Interesting point of view, I have this point of view. Interesting point of view, I have this point of view."

- "Interesting point of view, I have this judgment. Interesting point of view, I have this judgment. Interesting point of view, I have this judgment."

Using this tool allows the fixed points of view that are creating the limitation of judgment to unravel and dissipate.

Destroying and Un-creating Judgment

Judgment is insidious in the modern-day world and getting out of this limitation can be a process that takes time in its unfolding. We encourage you to keep practicing these tools. If you find yourself in judgment, you can always use the simplified clearing statement as previously mentioned.

Statements and questions for clearing judgments:

- "Everywhere I'm judging myself, I will now destroy and un-create it all."

- "Everywhere I'm judging my partner, I will now destroy and un-create it all."

- "Everywhere I have bought the judgments of others, I will now destroy and un-create them all."

- "Am I using judgment right now? If so, I will now destroy and un-create it all."

- "What else is possible beyond judgment?"

- "What am I grateful for?"

Creating a Relationship Beyond Judgment

As previously discussed, when creating a relationship beyond judgment, you are in allowance for the choices that you and your partner are making.

Many of us have learned to judge our partners about *everything*. We are often taught to have fixed points of view about who our partner should be, and then judge them if they don't conform to our expectations. Imagine what our world would be like if we no longer operated from judgment?

The following scenario shows the difference between the old paradigm of judgment and the new paradigm of putting these tools into action. Here, both partners have been strict vegetarians and one of the partners suddenly chooses to start eating meat.

In the old paradigm, the vegetarian partner goes into judgment, believes in the wrongness of their partner's new choice and says, "How could you eat meat! That's disgusting! It's bad for your body and we can't afford it." The other partner says, "It's my body, don't tell me what to do! Fine, I'll just eat in the other room on my own." The vegetarian states, "But you can't do that because we don't allow meat in our house!"

In the new paradigm, the vegetarian partner says, "That's an interesting choice that you are eating meat again." The other partner says, "I went to the grocery store and I asked my body, 'What other choices are available with food?' and I was instantly drawn to the meat section. Though I was surprised in that 10 seconds when I picked up the meat, I perceived that it was light and expansive for my body."

"Honey, I'm so happy you are trusting your awareness 10 seconds at a time and choosing what you know your body needs. I know the meat is a little more expensive, so what will it take for more money to show up for us?" The other says, "I'm very grateful you have so much allowance for my choices."

The tools in this book are designed to be pragmatic and easy to use in any situation. We encourage you to practice using them for creating your life and relationship beyond judgment.

Your Enjoyable Other

What if you could just immensely enjoy yourself and also enjoy your partner? This creates a space and freedom for both of you to just be yourselves and to create your relationship beyond judgment.

Calling your partner "my enjoyable other" is a fun, kind and playful way of referring to your partner.

Gratitude

Gratitude is an amazing gift and always creates something greater. When you are in gratitude, judgment cannot exist. And when you are grateful for yourself, it's a great starting place for being able to have gratitude for your partner. When you are grateful for your partner, there is no separation or judgment and this allows for the gratitude and love to grow.

Gratitude allows you to be grateful that your partner is in your life, and grateful for all the moments you're able to share together. Using gratitude and expanding your allowance are two of the many tools in this book for creating a relationship beyond judgment.

We invite you to use these tools with kindness and caring, while truly being in the question of "What else is possible?"

Summary of the Tools, Concepts and Questions from Chapter Six

1. "What's it going to take for more of *that* to show up?" — A question to ask when you desire more of something to show up in your life.

2. "Is this a judgment or an awareness?" — A question to ask when you need clarity as to whether you're having an awareness or a judgment.

3. "How does it get any better than this?" — A question to ask when things are going well, or not going well, to allow something greater to show up.

4. "What else is possible?" — A question for opening the door to new possibilities in every situation of your life and relationship.

5. Wearing rose-colored glasses — A well-known expression for how we use a filtering system of judgment for seeing things as we would like them to be, rather than as they are.

We know that creating a relationship beyond judgment is a big topic and we encourage you to practice using these tools daily. Undoing judgments is a process that unfolds, so please be kind to yourself and know that every 10 seconds you have a new choice. If you find yourself in judgment, in the next 10 seconds you can always choose something different. How does it get any better than this?

Much of what we have looked at so far revolves around using the tools to expand your awareness. A big part of expanding your awareness also includes the body. In the next chapter we will explore the body, and the role it plays in your life and relationship.

CHAPTER SEVEN

A New Kind of Relationship with Your Body

~

OUR BODIES ARE amazing sensory awareness organisms that are constantly giving us information. The tools presented throughout this book guide you on how to use this awareness for creating the life, body and relationship that you *really* desire. Imagine being empowered to experience enjoyment and pleasure with your body, no matter what you're doing.

In the new paradigm, while learning the language of your body, you increase the quality of living, where infinite possibilities of nurturing and caring are available to you. And this, of course, includes ways you can contribute to your partner's body. In this chapter we're going to explore new and enjoyable ways in which the body comes into play in your relationship.

What is Your Body Really?

The body is scientifically proven to be 99.996% empty space. If you took away the empty space that is between the atoms, and pushed them together, a person's body would be compressed to about the size of a pea.

Since atoms make up the entire body and are also mostly empty space, if you pushed them together until the nuclei were touching, then the body would be too small to see. If space were eliminated from all bodies and the matter was condensed, the entire population on Earth would fit into something like the size of a sugar cube.

Nobel Prize-winning physicists have proven that the physical world and our bodies are comprised of energy and that nothing is solid. Our five physical senses of sight, hearing, touch, smell, and taste are how we perceive this energy, and our thoughts determine the form this energy takes. In other words, our thoughts and points of view are what create our reality in the physical world.

The body is a sensory awareness organism and as such, has a consciousness of its own. When you learn to listen to your body's innate wisdom, it can contribute greatly to every area of your life. In this new kind of relationship with your body, the body is acknowledged as being comprised of energy, space, and consciousness and this opens a door to new possibilities.

Creating Your Body Beyond Judgment

The body is an amazing gift and in the new paradigm you are empowered to create your body beyond judgment. As young children, many of us had a lot of sexual energy and we explored, played and touched our bodies without having any judgment of whether it was right or wrong. What if we could still have this same kind of playfulness and ease with our bodies?

We start out as sexual beings — part of our natural way of being — and then we begin to get a downpour of other people's judgments that starts to diminish our sexual energy. Many people have learned to replace their sexual awareness with judgment.

In the old paradigm, our natural "sexualness" is overridden by judging our bodies and treating them poorly. For many people, if they treated their dog in the way they treat their bodies, their dog would run away. Have you noticed how many people take better care of their cars than they do of their bodies?

When you create your body beyond judgment, you allow your natural "sexualness" to flow. Sexualness is the energy of living and what you perceive in nature, where there is no judgment. It is the nurturing, caring, healing, creative, exciting, expansive, joyful, and orgasmic quality of living.

Questions and clearings for undoing judgments about the body:

The next time you find yourself in judgment of your body, you can ask:

- "Is this judgment really mine?"

- "Who does this judgment belong to?"

- "What other choices can I make in the next 10 seconds?"

- "All the judgments I have of my body, I will now destroy and un-create them all."

If you had no judgment of your body, what would your body say to you?

If you had no judgment of your body, what would you say to your body?

What else is possible with taking care of your body that you have never considered before?

Your Body as a Tool for Receiving Awareness

All along in this book, we have been introducing many tool and concepts. In this chapter, we're going to revisit some of them, as they relate to the body.

Light and Heavy

As previously highlighted, perceiving the energy of *your* light or heavy is about becoming aware of your body's sensations. In the old paradigm, these sensations are often called 'feelings' and what we're expanding upon here is empowering you to perceive the awareness that your body is giving you.

Using the tool of Perceiving Your Light and Heavy is a way of including your body in the choices you make and choosing from a place of expansion and possibility, rather than from contraction and conclusion. The more aware you are of the information your body gives you by perceiving what's light or heavy for you, the easier it becomes to make choices that work for you, and to be aware of what those choices will create.

Here's an example of how light and heavy applies to the body. Let's say you go to the gym and start training with a personal trainer. The trainer tells you to do a specific exercise, yet your awareness is that it's really heavy to do the exercise and your body is saying, "No! Don't do this." You ignore the awareness your body is giving you and do the exercise anyway and subsequently you injure your body.

Let's say on another day at the gym, as you go to use a certain machine, you get an awareness from your body that it's heavy for you to use the machine, so you choose not to. Shortly thereafter, someone else uses that same machine and it malfunctions, injuring that person.

Let's say you normally go to the gym every Monday. On one particular Monday, right before you head to the gym, a friend calls you and invites you to a cocktail party. The awareness of attending this party is so light and expansive that you choose to go there, rather than the gym. At the party, you meet an amazing person that ends up becoming your enjoyable other.

These are examples of Perceiving Your Light and Heavy and learning to follow your own awareness.

Have you ever had something wonderful show up for your body from a choice that you knew was the correct choice for you, even though everyone else discouraged you from choosing it? When you choose what you know is light and expansive for your body, it always creates something greater than anyone else's conclusion about what's right for your body.

10-Second Increments

We've talked a lot in this book about knowing what does and doesn't work for you and making choices in 10-second increments. What's light and works for you in one 10 seconds may not be light or work for you in the next 10 seconds. When you are in question with your body, in 10-second increments, you start to open up a whole new set of possibilities for the enjoyment of your body.

Let's say you take a walk every day and go on the same route and one day your body gives you the awareness that it desires to go in a different direction. Though this doesn't make any cognitive sense to you, you perceive that it's light and expansive, so you do it. Halfway along this new route, you see something shiny, you pick it up, and it's an antique gold coin.

Following your awareness of what's light and expansive for you, though it seldom shows up as you imagined, is part of the adventure and joy of living without limits.

Allowance

The more you pay attention to the information that your body is giving you, the more aware you become. As you become more aware, you may find that you need to expand your allowance to not be overwhelmed by all this new awareness you're receiving. You can ask, "Has my awareness exceeded my allowance?" If it's light and expansive when you ask this question, then this is true for you, so you can ask for your allowance to expand.

Vulnerability

Vulnerability is a strength and a way of having a deeper connection and more intimacy with your body and other bodies. By lowering your barriers, you can choose to be totally vulnerable with others in your life, and this becomes an invitation for them to lower their barriers and also be vulnerable. When you perceive that you have barriers up, you can ask for them to lower or just energetically push them down.

"Who Does This Belong To?"

Now, let's see how the tool of "Who Does This Belong To?" can be applied to the awareness of your body.

Let's say you're having a great day, and all of a sudden you start feeling really depressed. So you ask, "Who does this belong to?" The depressed feeling goes away and you're feeling great again.

Here are two more examples: Gary Douglas and Dain Heer were in Sydney many years ago and Dain asked Gary if he wanted to go eat sushi. Gary said, "I don't eat sushi." Dain asked, "Whose point of view is that?" Gary replied, "Not mine!" They immediately went and had sushi and Gary's been eating sushi ever since.

There was a woman who came to see Gary for facilitation around changing her body weight. After she was asked how many other people she was eating for, she realized that she had been picking up on everyone else's thoughts in the office about wanting to eat doughnuts and thinking the thoughts were her own. Once she started using the tool of "Who Does This Belong To?", she stopped eating so many doughnuts and was able to lose 20 pounds.

"Is This Really Mine?"

As previously discussed, many of our points of view are part of our cultural and social conditioning. Also, our bodies as sensory awareness organisms are aware of other people's bodies and their points of view and judgments.

So, the next time you notice a 'pain' in your body, we invite you to ask, "Is this really mine?" If the pain dissipates or goes away, you know that it wasn't yours in the first place.

Also, the next time you find yourself having points of view about your body or your intimate relationship with your partner's body and they seem out of character or not yours, you can ask "Is this point of view really mine?"

Let's say you're really turned on and desire to have sex with your partner. You suddenly look in the mirror and think, "I'm so fat and undesirable." You return to the room where your partner is and start having thoughts going through your head that your partner could never be attracted to you because you're fat and undesirable. You stop and realize that your partner is wildly attracted to you and shows you this every day. At this moment, if you ask, "Is this my awareness of someone else's point of view?" or "Is this really mine?", most likely the judgments will dissipate and go away.

Interesting Point of View

Having an "interesting point of view", rather than a 'fixed point of view', regarding anything about your body or your partner's body is one of the greatest freedoms and joys you can have in your life and relationship.

The next time you have fixed points of view about your body, you can say three or more times, "Interesting point of view, I have this point of view about my body. Interesting point of view, I have this point of view about my body. Interesting point of view, I have this point of view about my body."

What Else is Possible?

"What else is possible?" is an awesome question you can ask about anything relating to your body or your partner's body. The next time you have a great accomplishment with your body, like completing a ten-mile hike, you can acknowledge this, and then ask, "What else is possible?" and see what else shows up. Also, when you have a challenge with your body, you can ask, "What else is possible?" and see what else beyond the challenges shows up.

New Tools for More Awareness with Your Body

Connecting with the Earth

Walking barefoot on the Earth and allowing the Earth to contribute to you and your body is a great way of getting present, relaxed, of unwinding and returning to the space of being you. This is also an activity that you can do with your partner.

Your body as a sensory awareness organism is giving you information about the Earth and the world around you. When you're perceiving all of this awareness of the Earth through your body, and you are feeling overwhelmed, you can ask, "Is this mine or is this my awareness of the Earth?" If it's your awareness of the Earth, and you acknowledge this, the overwhelm will most likely will dissipate.

NIRMADA: A friend of mine used to get a lot of migraine headaches. After she learned to ask questions and be more aware of the information her body was giving her, she realized she only got migraine headaches right before a significant earthquake. Once she realized her headaches were related to her awareness of the Earth, she was able to dissipate the headaches by asking questions and using the tool of "Who Does This Belong To? "

Another way to receive with your body and connect with the Earth is to ask, "Am I receiving from the Earth?" If you get that you're not receiving from the Earth, you can say, "Everywhere I'm not receiving from the Earth, I will now destroy and un-create it all."

Energy Flows

In the old paradigm, many of us learned to put up barriers and not receive. When somebody puts up a barrier to you, no matter what you say to them, they cannot receive it. There's an easy way, using "energy flows", to create a connection with this person, beyond their barriers.

How to Use Energy Flows

If your partner has their barriers up and isn't receiving from you, you can lower your barriers and start flowing massive amounts of energy from all directions through their body and then through *your* whole body until you feel a connection with your partner and your heart opens. Flowing the energy in this way allows you to create a connection with your partner and it can sometimes be easier than doing it from talking.

To flow energy, all you have to do is ask for it to flow and intend for it flow. When you flow energy, it's not cognitive and you might not feel it right away. However, you may become aware of a sense of expansion and space.

Lowering your barriers and pulling energy through your partner is also a way of getting your partner to lower their barriers. You can put this into practice when there is a conflict or your partner is angry. For instance, if your partner starts yelling at you, you can either put up your barriers and resist the energy or you can lower your barriers and allow it to pass right through you without being affected by it. This is a way of resolving conflicts quickly and easily.

AN EXERCISE IN EXPANDING YOUR ENERGY

Begin by expanding your energy in all directions to the edges of the room you're in. Now keep expanding your energy out further in all directions to the edges of the building you're in. Keep expanding your energy out further in all directions to the edges of the neighborhood you're in. Keep expanding your energy out one mile in all directions including down into the Earth. Now expand out 10 miles in all directions including down into the Earth. Now expand out 100 miles further in all directions including down into the Earth. Now expand out 1000 miles further in all directions. Now expand out 10,000 miles further in all directions. How does that feel? Do you have a greater sense of space? You can keep expanding out as far as you desire.

You can expand your energy out beyond the borders of your body, in all directions: in front of you, to the right of you, to the back of you, to the left of you, as well as up into the sky and down into the Earth. You can do this standing, sitting or lying down.

This exercise can be used anytime to expand your energy or awareness. It is not recommended to do this while driving.

Asking Questions Including Your Body

We have spoken quite a bit about undoing judgments and fixed points of view through asking questions. Now you can ask questions, opening the door to new possibilities, and include your body. You can receive awareness from your body by asking questions and perceiving the sensory awareness of light or heavy.

Below are examples of different ways you can ask questions that include your body so that you can learn your body's language.

Your Body and Food

If you didn't have a body, would you need to eat? Since you wouldn't need to eat if you didn't have a body, doesn't it make sense to ask your body what it would like to eat? In the old paradigm, we are taught to conclude what our body needs to eat, rather than asking our body what it desires to eat.

Some questions you can ask your body:

- "Body, what would you like to eat?"

- "Body, what would you like to drink?"

- "Who does this hunger belong to?"

- "Body, is this really *your* hunger?"

The next time that you're 'hungry', you can ask your body, "Body, do you require food, or something to drink, or a walk, or sex, or touch?" Perhaps you'll discover, through asking your body questions, that your body isn't really hungry and desires something else. This is one of the ways, in the new paradigm, of being kind, caring and nurturing to your body.

Your Body and Your Partner's Body

Getting to know your body and your partner's body through asking questions is a harmonious way of connecting and creating more intimacy with each other.

Questions you can ask regarding your body and your partner's body:

- "Body, how would you like to be touched by our enjoyable other?"

- "Body, how would our enjoyable other's body like to be touched?"

- "How can I use my body's awareness to know what my partner's body requires?"

- "Body, what would be fun for you to receive?"

Asking to receive what feels good for your body, and asking your partner's body what feels good for it to receive, is a kind and nurturing way of having fun and enjoying your bodies together.

Your Body and Movement

Being in question with your body and how it desires to move is a way of connecting with your body. In the old paradigm, there are so many conclusions about what's the right or wrong thing to do with your body. We recommend asking questions and allowing your body to guide you with what it desires.

When walking, notice how you're walking: are you in front of your body pulling it along, or are you behind your body pushing it along or are you moving through space *with* your body? By observing how other people move their bodies, you'll gain more awareness of how this works.

Bodies desire movement and many of us have been entrained to force our bodies to do all kinds of prescribed exercise routines, rather than asking our bodies what types of movement would be fun and enjoyable for them.

Your Body and Lovemaking

Lovemaking can be a fun and enjoyable movement for your body. You can ask your body if it would like to have sex, when it would like to have sex, and how often it would like to have sex. This is a way of honoring your body and learning to honor your partner's body. Sometimes your body may desire sex more than your partner's body, so asking questions and having allowance for whatever shows up will create more ease.

Your Body and Sleep

Many people conclude that they need a prescribed amount of sleep. What if, instead, you were to ask questions of your body and become aware of how much sleep your body actually requires.

Questions you can ask your body:

- "Body, how much sleep do you require?"

- "Body, are you tired or are you just aware of someone else's tiredness?"

Your body's sleep requirements may differ from day to day and may be different from your partner's body. Having allowance for the fluctuations in the sleep requirements of your body and those of your partner's body will create more harmony and ease.

AN EXERCISE IN BECOMING PRESENT WITH YOUR BODY

Connecting with the senses of your body is a way of getting present with your body. Either sitting or lying down, begin by closing your eyes and taking a deep breath in and, on the out breath, relax your whole body. Become aware of the weight of your body on the chair you are sitting on or the surface you're touching. Feel the gentle movement of air on your skin. Feel the weight of your clothes on your body. Connect with the taste in your mouth. Connect to the sounds that are closest to you and then allow your listening to expand out to the furthest sounds you can hear and remain there. After a few moments, come back to your body.

Are you now more present with your body?

Orgasmic Living

What if your life could be an orgasmic experience?

In the old paradigm, orgasm is often related to the outcome of sexual intercourse. In the new paradigm, orgasm is the energy of living without limits and contributes to the creation of your body. Orgasmic living includes the energy and sensations of being present and aware, whether you're walking barefoot on the Earth, eating food, reading a book, playing a sport or making love.

The tools presented in this book are here to guide you in having pleasure and enjoyment with your body and your partner's body, no matter what you're doing. When both of your bodies experience pleasure and joy, you begin to create your lives as orgasmic.

In the new paradigm, we acknowledge that bodies love to be touched and this doesn't necessarily mean it's about sex. The energy that we are referring to here is what we have called "sexualness". Sexualness is the energy of what you feel when you're in nature and where there's no judgment. It's the orgasmic quality of living and includes the energies that are nurturing, caring, healing, creative, expansive, joyful, and generative.

Receiving and Lovemaking in 10-Second Increments

We previously spoke about lovemaking in 10-second increments. This means taking the performance element out of sex and just enjoying each other's bodies in the moment. This removes judgments and expectations from your sexual experiences and allows you to experience the orgasmic quality of living without limits. When you're willing to connect with and receive your partner and their body without judgment, then you can easily share orgasmic living together.

What if every time you have sex it is more fun and enjoyable than you imagined?

AN EXERCISE IN MAKING OUT IN 10-SECOND INCREMENTS

We invite you to practice being present with your body and your partner's body by making out in 10-second increments. What we are suggesting here is to kiss with your partner for 10 seconds and then stop. Then kiss with your partner for another 10 seconds and then stop. Enjoy every 10 seconds of kissing as long as it's fun for you and your partner to continue this exercise.

Contributing to Your Partner's Body

In the new paradigm, contributing to your partner's body goes way beyond sex and physical affection. A great tool you can use to contribute to your partner is to ask, "What energy, space, and consciousness can my body be to contribute to your body with ease?" Then use your awareness of where to place your hands on your partner's body. This can be for as long or short a period as desired.

Another simple tool for working with your partner's body is to put your hands on their heart or the center of their chest and ask, "What can I contribute here?" Relax, allow the energy to flow and enjoy! Start practicing this in times when the connection between you is easy. You can also progress to doing this when there's a conflict or misunderstanding between you. In the new paradigm, when there's a conflict or an argument, you're invited to not put up barriers or withdraw your physical touch or contribution.

Sometimes contributing to your partner's body may require that you give them space. Also, we suggest being aware of when *you* require space and that you ask for what you require.

Gifting and Receiving With Your Bodies

Gifting and receiving simultaneously with your body and your partner's body is a great way of increasing your connectedness and orgasmic living. Receiving is one of our greatest capacities and one of the ways that so many people have cut off and learned to refuse dynamically.

One of the ways that we cut off our receiving is through functioning from thoughts, feelings and emotions, and then determining, judging and concluding what we can and can't receive. But nobody in the old paradigm is actually taught to receive.

As mentioned in the Introduction, most of the tools in this book have come from Access Consciousness. One of the hands-on tools for learning to receive is something called The Access Bars®; this is changing lives dynamically in almost 200 countries around the world.

The Bars are 32 points on the head where we've stored all the thoughts, ideas, beliefs, considerations and emotions that we thought were important. When you "get your Bars run", it's like hitting the delete button on a computer: it allows you to begin functioning from beyond the limitations of the old paradigm. Receiving

Bars is a pleasurable way to begin functioning from receiving.

Running Bars is easy to learn and a fun and delightful activity that you can enjoy and share with your partner. See *Resources* for learning more about the Access Bars.

NIRMADA: When I received Bars for the first time, it changed everything in my life. I started to feel so much calm and ease with my body and in my life. All the things I had bought as true started to dissipate and I realized that I had never fully received before I had my first Bars session. I'm so grateful for Bars as it continues to contribute to expanding every area of my life.

Acknowledgment and Gratitude For Your Body

Acknowledgment and gratitude are two of the tools that we've spoken about a lot in this book. When you practice having gratitude for your body, it's an easy way to begin living without limits. Your body will be with you for the rest of this life, so our question to you is, "How much fun and enjoyment can you have with *your* body?"

"Living Without Limits", as the subtitle suggests, is something that unfolds with each choice you make and 10 seconds at a time. So, would you consider acknowledging yourself and your body for wherever you're currently at on *your* journey of living without limits?

NIRMADA: Every day I do my best to acknowledge the things I have accomplished in the day that were greater than the day before. Sometimes I say them to myself and sometimes I'll say them when I'm having a conversation with John. It can be anything from doing a new exercise at the gym to accomplishing a creative project.

Summary of the Tools, Concepts and Questions from Chapter Seven

1. The body is a sensory awareness organism and has a consciousness of its own. When you learn to listen to your body's innate wisdom, it can contribute greatly to every area of your life.

2. In the new paradigm, contributing to your body and your partner's body goes way beyond sex and physical affection. A great tool you can use to contribute to your partner is to ask, "What energy, space, and

consciousness can my body be to contribute to your body with ease?"

3. Use the tool of Perceiving Your Light and Heavy for making choices by first becoming aware of your body's sensations and then listening to your body's light and heavy.

4. When you create your body beyond judgment, this allows your natural sexualness to flow.

5. Having an "interesting point of view" rather than a 'fixed point of view' regarding anything about your body or your partner's body is one of the greatest freedoms and joys you can have in your life and relationship.

6. "What else is possible?" is an awesome question you can ask for anything relating to your body or your partner's body.

7. Connecting with the Earth—Walking barefoot on the Earth and allowing the Earth to contribute to you and your body is a great way of getting present, relaxed, of unwinding and returning to the space of being you. This is also an activity that you can do with your partner.

8. Orgasmic Living—What if your life could be an orgasmic experience?

9. Access Bars is easy to learn and a fun and delightful activity that you can enjoy and share with your partner. See *Resources* for learning more about the Access Bars.

We've looked at the enjoyment of your body and some new ways you can explore it in your relationship. In the next chapter we'll begin to look at questions you can ask for changing your reality.

CHAPTER EIGHT

Asking Questions for Changing Your Reality

~

LOVE IN THE Next 10 Seconds was written for you, the reader, to know that you have choice every 10 seconds. When you apply the tools and questions in this book, you have the possibility for changing many areas of your life with ease.

When you are willing to ask questions, you can change anything. This enables you to create the ease of an orgasmic quality of living, where your reality includes the generative energies that are nurturing, caring, healing, creative, expansive and joyful.

Would You Rather Be Right or Would You Rather Be Free?

The tools and questions explored in this chapter will enable you to navigate your way with ease through conflicts and change in any area of your life.

As mentioned before, many conflicts in the old paradigm are created from having a 'somebody is right or wrong' fixed point of view and when this happens, it becomes a challenge to change the situation. When you get out of having fixed points of view and into asking questions, you can change many situations with ease.

Whenever you find yourself defending the rightness of your point of view, you can ask yourself: "Would I rather be right or would I rather be free?" Asking this question creates more freedom in your life and relationship. Remember, when you ask questions, you are not looking for an answer; you are, instead, open to receiving more awareness. The willingness to let go of your fixed points of view and asking questions will create change.

When your partner says or does something that you don't like, you may have learned to make a blaming statement like "You just really hurt me!" Now, instead of putting your partner on the defensive, you can open up the possibilities for changing the situation by asking the question, "What did you intend by that?" When you ask a question like this, it allows you and your partner to harmoniously communicate for changing the situation with ease.

When both partners are defending the rightness of their points of view, it can become the perfect storm for creating a conflict. Saying the simple statement "You are right and I am wrong," three or more times can quickly and easily undo a conflict. It's not relevant who is right or wrong; what's important is that you are capable of changing the situation and having the freedom to enjoy and create your life.

What's it Going to Take to Change This?

In the new paradigm, you are encouraged to be empowered to use your awareness, questions and these tools for changing any area of your life that isn't working for you.

Two questions you can ask as a way of changing many situations are: "What will it take to change this?" or "What else can I be or do today to change this right away?" Here are some practical ways you can apply these questions in your everyday life.

Let's say your partner comes home in a really bad mood and starts complaining about how little money they have. You could conclude that this is the way it is, or you could ask your partner: "What will it take to change your financial reality?" If your partner were to reply, "I have no idea what it would take to change this," you could then ask: "What else could you be or do today to have more money show up right away?"

You can then reassure your partner that it's okay to allow the awareness from these questions to come to them, and that it's not necessary to look for the answers. You can also apply these questions to changing any area of your own life.

What's Right about This That I'm Not Getting?

What if you could allow every experience in your life to contribute to you, regardless of the outcome? When things don't show up like you imagined they would, or when things appear to be mishaps, rather than concluding "I can't believe this just happened!", you could ask: "What's right about this that I'm not getting?"

When you get out of judging your choices and life experiences as 'right or wrong' or 'good or bad', you allow yourself to expand to a new level of freedom, joy and possibility. This means that you are willing to use any experience in your life to gain more awareness, which then opens the door to new possibilities. When you are welcoming awareness, even when it is uncomfortable, it expands your reality and is the ultimate in receiving new possibilities.

When you are judging yourself, a quick way of changing this is to ask: "What's right about me that I'm not getting?" Asking this question can shift your perspective away from wrongness and open you up to new ways of seeing things.

What Else Can I Be or Do Today to Change This?

As we have mentioned, asking "What else can I be or do today to change this right away?" is a great question to ask when you desire something to change. When you ask this question, you may not receive the awareness right away. Things rarely show up like you imagined, so be open to the awareness coming from anywhere for what it's going to take to change it.

Here are some fun ways of using this question:

- "What else can I be or do today to have more fun with my partner right away?"

- "What else can I be or do today to have more intimacy with my partner right away?"

- "What else can I be or do today to improve my relationship right away?"

Four Questions to Change Anything

These four questions are a great way to navigate your way to change with any situation that shows up. When you require something to change, you can ask these four questions of the situation:

- "What is this?"

- "What do I do with it?"

- "Can I change it?"

- "And if so, how can I change it?"

We will explore these four questions a little more deeply, so you can see how to apply them to everyday situations.

- **What is this?**

When you ask this question of a situation, you are asking for the awareness of what is beyond anything you've already concluded it is. Remember, the awareness may not come right away or in the form you were expecting.

- **What do I do with it?**

After asking this question, allow the awareness to come to you when and how it does.

- **Can I change it?**

Sometimes you may get the awareness that you can change the situation and sometimes you will get the awareness that you can't change it. If you get a 'yes' (you can change it), then you can go on to ask the fourth question. If you get a 'no' (you can't change it), just remember to have allowance and continue to receive the awareness from asking the previous two questions.

- **How do I change it?**

Sometimes you may get the awareness right away on how to change the situation and sometimes you will get the awareness later. The key in asking these questions is that you are open to new possibilities that can show up to change things beyond what you have imagined.

And when you get a 'no', indicating you can't change something, rather than concluding that it's wrong, ask "What else is possible?" or "How does it get any better than this?" These questions create something greater when things are going well and also when things aren't going well and require changing.

Adding To, Rather than Getting Rid Of

As soon as you notice that something is not working, you can approach it with curiosity in order to create space for it to change. You don't have to find a fault or get rid of anything in order for it to change. Instead, you can ask, "What can I add to my life today to have more _____ right away?"

Let's say that you got a huge electricity bill that you weren't expecting. You might go into reaction mode and start looking into all the areas where you need to cut your expenses. Alternatively, you could ask, "What can I add to my life today to create more money right away?" By asking this question you open yourself up to receiving awareness for new ways of creating money.

When you are willing to add to your life, you give yourself a way to expand and create your reality. Here are some other ways you can use this question:

- "What can I add to my life today to have more joy right away?"

- "What can I add to my life today to have greater health right away?"

- "What can I add to my life today to have a better relationship right away?"

NIRMADA: I knew I desired to make some changes with my body, so I started asking, "What can I add to my life today to change my body right away?" After a few days of asking this question, I met a friend of a friend that was a personal trainer and I started training with them. Amazing changes are being created with my body from the training sessions.

What Other Choices are Available?

When things don't show up as we have imagined, we can sometimes create a situation where we go into limitation and conclusion. Whenever you find yourself going into a situation where you believe it's the only choice you have, you can ask, "What other choices are available that I haven't yet considered?"

When you ask this question, it changes the situation and allows you to have more choices available than you had previously considered.

NIRMADA: One time, John and I went to a hotel and we were told that there were no more rooms available. We requested to speak with the manager and asked, "What other choices are available?" The manager kept on looking and finally said, "I have one executive suite available that I will give to you at the regular room rate." Asking this question opened the door to receiving an amazing room and with a complimentary upgrade.

The Difference between Advice and Facilitation

Your own awareness is more powerful than anyone else's answers. Being empowered to know what you know is a way of honoring yourself and others. Trusting your awareness includes knowing when you require, or your partner requires, someone else's contribution or facilitation.

Many people in relationship seek outside advice when there are challenges. Advice, in the old paradigm, could be loosely defined as other people's projections, opinions and points of view about your relationship.

Advice sometimes helps and sometimes it can do the opposite. With good quality facilitation, where someone asks you questions, you are empowered to navigate your way to becoming more aware of the situation and to see what it's going to take to change it.

If you are new to asking questions or changing things on your own, it can be useful to receive facilitation from someone who is experienced in asking questions for changing things. This is very different from counseling or getting advice.

Facilitation is about empowering you to know what you know, through asking questions, and this enables you to receive more awareness. As your awareness increases, you will expand the array of choices that are available to you.

How different is this to being told who you should be and what you should do?

Suggestions on How to Facilitate Your Partner

Do you know someone who has no judgment of you? How wonderful is it to be around this kindness and caring? It is this kindness and caring that you can use to facilitate your partner (or anyone else for that matter). Having no judgment in facilitation means that you have an "interesting point a view" about whatever is being said.

We suggest that you don't start facilitating your partner unless they have asked you for facilitation. However, the following questions can open up the possibilities for this:

- "Can I ask you a question?"

- "Can I contribute anything to you?"

- "Do you require some facilitation?"

NIRMADA: We only facilitate each other when one of us asks for it or we have permission. Sometimes one of us will ask the other for facilitation and sometimes one of us will ask the other if they require facilitation.

JOHN: Recently, when Nirmada asked me if there was anything that she could contribute to me for changing what was going on, I asked her, "How expanded are you right now?" She replied, "Very expanded." I replied, "Can you just be that expanded energy rather than saying anything, and allow that to contribute to me?"

Being in Nirmada's expanded presence was exactly the kind of support that I required in that moment. She was in allowance and honoring the space that I required.

We invite you to have fun with facilitating your partner or being facilitated by your partner. For example, you could go for a walk in nature and then ask your partner to facilitate you. Also, while lying in bed at night, you and your partner could have a nightly ritual of facilitating and contributing to each other. Having allowance for your partner's choices and asking questions in a kind and caring way create more intimacy together as you contribute to each other.

Asking Questions vs. Giving Answers

The following table shows the difference between facilitating through asking questions and possibility, and giving answers and conclusions.

The column on the left presents some of the possibilities of the new paradigm. The column on the right presents some of the limitations of the old paradigm. As you look over this table, we invite you to perceive your **light** and **heavy** as you compare the words in both columns.

Choice	Conclusion
Question	Answer
Possibility	Expectation
Contributing	Taking
Infinite	Finite
Interesting point of view	This is right. This is wrong.
What other choices are available?	I must do this. I have to do this.
What would I like to create?	What do I need to do?
Neutrality	Polarity
The Kingdom of We	The Kingdom of Me
Gratitude	Judgment
What can they receive?	I have decided you need this.
What else is possible?	Fixed points of view, conclusion
Energy, space and consciousness	Time, matter, limitation
What can I be or do to change this?	What must I do to fix this?
Spaciousness	Density
Limitless	Limited

This table is here to empower you to become aware of the infinite choices you have available to you, in every 10 seconds.

Creating Beyond the Invention of Problems

Have you ever encountered someone who perceived they had a problem, yet it was really obvious to you that it was made up in their mind and something they had invented? Many so-called 'problems' that we experience are actually inventions and aren't real, even if they seem as though they are real at the time.

Perhaps you can look back at something from your past that you were convinced was an issue. When you reflect on it now, can you see that you were temporarily convinced by a belief that the problem was real, even when it wasn't? Many conflicts in relationship often begin with the invention of a problem, and the tools in this book will enable you to change this in a kind and caring way.

One way of undoing an upset is to ask yourself, or your partner, in a kind way, "Is this *really* a problem or is it an invention?" Oftentimes, the invention of a problem can overshadow the caring of each other. Traditionally, in the old paradigm, a 'problem' can create separation between partners, taking them out of The Kingdom of We and into The Kingdom of Me.

NIRMADA: One night, when John and I were getting to know each other, I had a big meltdown about our relationship. I was really uncomfortable and had invented that it was over between us. John very kindly facilitated me until the invented problems and fixed points of view dissipated.

If we had concluded that things were not going to work, and he had not asked questions, we might have ended our relationship right then. By using the tools presented in this book, we were able to move beyond the invented problems and create an enormous amount of freedom and expansion in our lives and relationship.

Part of being empowered is first to acknowledge that you have invented a problem. An easy way to clear invented problems is to ask one of the questions below, following it up with the simplified clearing statement.

- "What invention am I using to create the upset I am choosing? Everything that is, I will now destroy and un-create it all."

- "What invention am I using to create the problem I am choosing? Everything that is, I will now destroy and un-create it all."

Once you realize you have created an upset in your relationship through an invention, an easy way to change the situation with your partner is to say, "I apologize. How can I make up for the damage done?" This level of vulnerability and kindness is part of living The Five Elements of Intimacy.

Throwing the Baby Out with the Bathwater

You might have heard the expression: "Don't throw the baby out with the bathwater". When something needs to change, particularly in relationships, rather than choosing 10 seconds at a time, many of us take an 'all or nothing' approach.

Have you ever been in an argument with your partner and abruptly concluded: "This isn't working! I'm out of here!" What if a different possibility were available when things get uncomfortable? When you are choosing in 10-second increments and asking questions, you open up the door to a new set of possibilities, regardless of the circumstances.

Two questions you can ask to change the dynamics of many situations are "What else is possible?" and "What's it going to take to change this?" The awareness that you will gain from asking these questions may come to you in any form and at any time. When you are willing to acknowledge what you are aware of, without the point of view that it is right or wrong, your freedom of choice begins.

Part of being aware is acknowledging when certain essential things in your relationship aren't working for you. You may be able to change some of these things in your relationship and there may be some things that you cannot change. Being clear about what does and doesn't work for you and making choices based on your awareness is "Changing the Box of Relationship Into Living Without Limits".

Being Comfortable with Being Uncomfortable

Being empowered means that you are the creator of your own reality. When you are the leader in your own life, you make choices that are not always easy. When you are following your awareness in 10-second increments, you choose what works for you and what you desire, regardless of how uncomfortable it is.

Change can often bring about a certain amount of discomfort. When you are uncomfortable, you can actually be grateful, because it means things are changing! Oftentimes the discomfort of change comes because your reality has become unfamiliar and undefined.

How many of us have learned to define our lives and relationship through conclusions and referring to past experiences? If you can be in allowance of this temporary discomfort, rather than resisting it, things can start to change.

NIRMADA AND JOHN: When we first started using the tools in this book and navigating change in our relationship, it was like we were out on the skinny branches. We were so uncomfortable, as the solidity of our lives, relationship, and realities began to dissolve. Over time, we have discovered that by learning to be comfortable with being uncomfortable, we have created a level of change and freedom that is beyond what we considered possible.

Some questions for creating more ease with change:

- "What will it take for me to be comfortable with being uncomfortable?"

- "What's it going to take to have more ease with this change?"

- "What can I be or do today to change this with ease right away?"

When you learn to be comfortable with being uncomfortable, you allow yourself and your relationship to enjoy the change that you are asking for.

When things are changing and it gets 'wonky' in your life or relationship, you can ask, "Is this the change I have been asking for?" or "Is this the change I have been asking for and it looks different than what I imagined?"

Acknowledgment and Gratitude

Acknowledgment and Gratitude are tools we mention a lot in this book and they can be used and enjoyed on a daily basis. As you apply the tools in this book, a lot of change will be created. We invite you to acknowledge yourself and to be grateful to yourself for having read this book up until now and for choosing to create something different.

- What are three things you can be grateful for about yourself?

- What are three things you can acknowledge about yourself?

- What are three things you have already changed that you can acknowledge and be grateful for?

We acknowledge you, the reader, for having the courage to follow your knowing and for creating your new paradigm of living without limits.

Summary of the Tools, Concepts and Questions from Chapter Eight

1. "Would I rather be right or would I rather be free?" — A question you can ask to create more freedom in your life and relationship.

2. "What's it going to take to change this?" and "What else can I be or do today to change this right away?" — Questions you can ask to get out of conclusions and into possibilities for changing many situations.

3. "What's right about this that I'm not getting?" — A question for receiving the contribution from your experiences, regardless of the outcome.

4. Four questions to navigate your way to changing anything:

    • "What is this?"

    • "What do I do with it?"

    • "Can I change it?"

    • "And if so, how can I change it?"

5. "What can I add to my life today to have more _____ right away?" — A question you can ask to get out of limitation and into creation mode.

6. "What other choices are available that I haven't yet considered?" — A question to open the door to more choices than you considered possible.

7. Questions you can ask to facilitate and empower your partner:

    • "Can I ask you a question?"

    • "Can I contribute anything to you?"

    • "Do you require some facilitation?"

8. Questions and clearings for undoing the invention of problems in your relationship:

   - "What invention am I using to create the upset I am choosing? Everything that is, I will now destroy and un-create it all."

   - "What invention am I using to create the problem I am choosing? Everything that is, I will now destroy and un-create it all."

9. "What else is possible?" and "What's it going to take to change this?" — Questions to create more possibility in any situation.

10. Questions for creating more ease with change:

    - "What will it take for me to be comfortable with being uncomfortable?"

    - "What's it going to take to have more ease with this change?"

    - "What else can I be or do today to change this with ease right away?"

11. "Is this the change I have been asking for?" or "Is this the change I have been asking for and it looks different than what I imagined?" — Questions

you can ask when things are changing and it gets 'wonky' in your life or relationship.

12. Questions you can ask to have more gratitude and acknowledgment in your life and relationship:

- "What are three things I can be grateful for about myself?"

- "What are three things I can acknowledge about myself?"

- "What are three things I have already changed that I can acknowledge and be grateful for?"

Having explored how to use these tools and questions pragmatically in your relationship, in Part Three of this book, we will be focusing on creating a relationship that you really desire. This includes gifting and receiving in your life and relationship, deepening your acknowledgment of one another and creating a world together that you both desire to live in.

PART THREE

Creating The Future You Really Desire

CHAPTER NINE

Gifting and Receiving in The New Paradigm

~

"Receiving is the ultimate in possibility." Gary Douglas

WHAT IF GIFTING and receiving with your partner could be as easy as breathing? When you gift and receive simultaneously with your partner, you open up the space for both of you to contribute to each other, and this creates new possibilities in your relationship.

The willingness to gift and receive simultaneously allows you to create your life and relationship beyond the 'exchange rate' of the old paradigm. In the new paradigm, you begin to acknowledge that when you are gifting, you are also receiving and when you are receiving, you are also gifting.

Have you ever gifted a present to someone that you cared about and they received it joyously in a way that made you feel really good? This is one of many ways you may experience gifting and receiving simultaneously. The following are additional examples of how this works.

Have you ever given money to a beggar and they said, "Thank you so much!" with a huge level of gratitude, and you received in a way that brightened up the rest of your day?

When you walk in nature, the plants, trees, animals and Earth are continuously gifting to you, and when you allow yourself to simultaneously receive it, it's a contribution and a gift to you. Have you noticed how nature gifts to you without expecting anything in return?

Have you ever experienced a communion with an animal, where the animal loved you without expecting anything in return, and it became a mutual gifting and receiving? This is an example of gifting and receiving beyond the expectations and 'exchange rate' of the old paradigm.

NIRMADA AND JOHN: When we first met in Costa Rica and were running energy on each other's body, there was a wonderful gifting and receiving between us. It was as though the whole world disappeared, and there was no time: there was just energy, space, and consciousness. This level of gifting and receiving with each other opened up the door for us to write *Love in the Next 10 Seconds* later on.

AN EXERCISE IN GIFTING AND RECEIVING WITH YOUR PARTNER

A simple way to practice gifting and receiving with your partner is to lay your hands on your partner's body at their heart center. First, notice your body's energy contributing to their body. Then notice your partner receiving the energy you are gifting to them and allow yourself to simultaneously receive the energy.

Gifting and Receiving with Acknowledgment

Acknowledgment is a tool that you can use regardless of what is going on in your relationship. Whether you are having a great day or a challenging day, acknowledgment will allow you to create something greater. When you use acknowledgment, you contribute to the expansion of gifting and receiving.

JOHN: One of the things I appreciate about Nirmada is that she will ask me, "Can I acknowledge you for something?" She regularly acknowledges me for being who I am and for how much I contribute to her life. I always expand and become lighter from receiving these acknowledgments.

NIRMADA: When there is a conflict between us, it is quickly dissipated by pausing and acknowledging what we are grateful for. I will ask John, "What are three things that you are grateful for?", and he will ask me the same. We acknowledge everything from how beautiful the day is, to how grateful we are to be in each other's life, for creating together, and for walking bare-foot on the Earth.

The Kingdom of We

In the new paradigm of gifting and receiving, it's about creating beyond the need to give something and then expecting to get something directly in return. In this way, gifting and receiving in relationship doesn't have an exchange rate.

Rather, it's a way of treating yourself and your partner with regard, and a willingness to gift and receive from The Kingdom of We. When you expand your awareness and choices to include what is good for yourself and your partner, then you are making choices based on The Kingdom of We.

Treating Your Partner with Regard when Gifting and Receiving

Treating your partner with regard when gifting and receiving is about being aware of what they are capable of receiving, and gifting them only that. Sometimes, you may see the possibilities of what your partner can be, even if they are unable to see it for themselves in that 10 seconds. They may not be ready to choose what you know is possible for them, and it's not a kindness to try to make them do so.

Seeing what they could be, or choose, doesn't mean that they will see it or choose it for themselves. True kindness is allowing your partner to choose what *they* desire and gifting to them only what they are able to receive.

When you do this, it's also showing true kindness to yourself. When you give someone more than they are capable of receiving, they can end up resisting it and then resenting you. When you allow yourself to be aware of what both of you are capable of receiving, it creates more harmony and ease in the relationship.

Questions to ask for gaining more awareness:

- "What will it take for me to be aware of what my partner can receive?"

- "What do I desire to receive?"

- "What can I receive beyond what I imagined possible?"

NIRMADA: It's my nature to desire that everyone receive everything I know they are capable of. What I came to realize was that I had be totally aware of what people could hear and receive and give them only that. It has been one of my big life lessons to recognize that just because I know something is possible, that doesn't mean that other people will see it or choose it.

JOHN: When I had my hands-on healing practice some years ago, I desired my clients to receive everything I had to offer. After years of trying to give people more than what they could receive, and making myself wrong when they couldn't receive it, I finally realized I could be aware of what they were capable of receiving and give them only that.

Gifting and Receiving with The Five Elements of Intimacy

Previously we explored **The Five Elements of Intimacy**, which are: Honor, Trust, Vulnerability, Allowance and Gratitude.

When you are honoring your partner, you have total regard and allowance for the choices that your partner makes. These choices include how much they are willing to gift and receive, regardless of the fact that you may know that they could choose something greater.

When we let our points of view determine what our partner should choose, we are not necessarily honoring them. Have you ever experienced someone who decided you needed to receive something when you had absolutely no desire for it? Perhaps you have had a partner or friend who went to a course or learned something new, and then projected their new perspective onto you with no regard as to whether you were interested in hearing about it or not.

What if, instead, you could ask your partner questions about what they desire to receive, which then allows them to get the awareness for themselves? The target is to keep asking questions, rather than thinking you have the answers or know what is right for your partner. And when you honor what works for your partner, remember to also honor what works for you.

Trust in the new paradigm is based on using your awareness to know what's true for you, 10 seconds at a time. What's true for you in this 10 seconds may not be true for you in the next 10 seconds. Trust includes being aware of what your partner can receive and also knowing what you desire to receive.

Vulnerability creates more intimacy with yourself and your partner. True receiving is when you allow yourself to be vulnerable with your barriers down and are willing to receive everything around you, without a point of view. Vulnerability is a strength that can be used to receive more of anything that you are asking for to show up in your life.

NIRMADA: When John and I first met, it was remarkable how vulnerable we were with each other and how much this contributed to our simultaneously gifting and receiving with each other.

JOHN: When we first met, I was so received by Nirmada that I could be totally open with her and talk about anything. It made it easy to be vulnerable and have my barriers lowered with her because she wasn't judging me and she was also being vulnerable.

When you are vulnerable and have your barriers lowered, it creates a whole different possibility for awareness and a new level of gifting and receiving with your partner. For instance, if your partner yells at you and you put up barriers, the intensity of their yelling will most likely increase, as they will attempt to knock the barriers down. Instead, if you lower your barriers, there will be no barriers for them to push against and this will most likely get them to stop yelling at you.

To lower your barriers, first ask for your barriers to lower and intend for them to lower. Then imagine pulling energy through the universe, through your partner and then through you. Keep doing this until your partner has also lowered their barriers and you both have a sense of peace and oneness.

Having allowance for the gifting and receiving your partner is capable of enables you to get out of making conclusions about what your relationship is supposed to be, and allows you to create it with ease, 10 seconds at a time. Whenever you find yourself becoming irritated or annoyed, remember that you can expand your allowance.

What if you could practice being grateful for everything that you and your partner gift to each other and receive from each other? When you are grateful for what you receive, you can ask, "How does it get any better than this?" and "What else is possible?" When you ask these questions your receiving continues to expand.

Questions for expanding gratitude:

- "What am I grateful for today?"

- "What am I grateful for about me?"

- "What am I grateful for about my partner?"

Gifting and Receiving with the World

Gifting and receiving includes the amazing contribution you are to the World. Have you acknowledged that you are a gift to the World? Many of us are not taught to see ourselves as a gift.

If you aren't sure what your gifts are yet, you can ask, "What is so easy for me to do that I don't even know it's a gift?" What talents or things come so naturally to you, that you may not have acknowledged them as your gifts to the world?

Questions and clearings for acknowledging your gifts:

- "What's so easy for me to do that I don't even know it's a gift?"

- "What are three of my gifts that I can acknowledge?"

- "What are three of my gifts that I am grateful for?"

- "Anything that doesn't allow me to know what my gifts are, I will now destroy and un-create it all."

NIRMADA AND JOHN: Gifting to the World is creating the kind of World that we would like to live in. This book is one of the ways that we are sharing our gifts with you and the World. It is not just about contributing to you so that you can have a more dynamic relationship. It is also about empowering you to be all that you can be, for living without limits.

Generosity of Spirit

True generosity of spirit is desiring everybody to receive everything they can, and being happy for them when they receive it. If you were to win the lottery tomorrow, how many people do you know who would be truly happy for you? The people who would be truly happy for you are the ones that have generosity of spirit.

When you are functioning from The Kingdom of We, you are embodying generosity of spirit. When you choose to be more conscious in your life and create a more conscious relationship, this contributes to everybody and is generosity of spirit. When people are happy that you have an awesome relationship—this is also generosity of spirit. What if you could practice celebrating every time someone you know receives something phenomenal?

Generosity of spirit includes being generous with yourself. Being generous with yourself is having allowance for where you are currently at, without making yourself wrong, and knowing you can choose something new in the next 10 seconds.

Gifting and Receiving with Your Body

Gifting and receiving with your body and your partner's body is a wonderful way of connecting. If you rub your partner's back, for example, you can perceive the energy of your gifting to them, while simultaneously receiving it. When you and your partner nurture each other's body, play with perceiving the energy of simultaneously gifting and receiving.

Perceiving energy is a muscle you build. Some people are able to perceive energy and for other people, it takes some practice. Be kind and patient with yourself and allow yourself to get it when you get it. When Gary created the Access Bars 25 years ago, he wasn't able to perceive energy. Over time this changed, and for two decades he has taught many people worldwide how to perceive energy.

Gifting and Receiving with Your Sexual Energy

How many of us in relationship have been entrained to believe that it is wrong to share our sexual energy with anyone other than our partner? How much receiving do you have to cut off by limiting yourself or your partner from expressing your sexual energies? We are not talking about the act of sexual intercourse—what we are describing here is you being all of you, and freely expressing yourself.

NIRMADA: Our willingness to be all of our sexual energy in any situation always creates something greater for both of us. One day, I came back from the store and told John that a guy I was standing next to in line totally turned my body on. There was nothing I had to do with this energy other than to receive it and enjoy it. John was so happy to receive the energy of my excitement and it was also a gift to him.

John has a great physique. When we are around other people we know, I will say things like "Doesn't John have a great ass?" I know I don't have to energetically keep him to myself or hold on to him tightly, and that other people can enjoy and appreciate his form too.

JOHN: When we are driving together down the street, quite often I will see someone really attractive and say, "That person has a really nice body!" Nirmada will always appreciate me admiring another body and always receives it as a contribution to her body.

When we cut off our sexual energy, we also cut off a lot of nurturing and generative energy.

- What if your sexual energy and your partner's sexual energy could be a gift to each other and to the World?

- What if your gifting and receiving of sexual energy and your partner's gifting and receiving of sexual energy were healing energies that created your new paradigm in relationship?

- And when your partner gifts their admiration to someone else, could you see this as a contribution to you and your relationship?

Receiving at this level ignites living The Five Elements of Intimacy. We highly recommend that when you and your partner practice gifting and receiving with your sexual energy that you do it through The Kingdom of We.

Have you ever considered the possibility that if you require your partner to cut off their sexual energy towards others that this also means they cut off their sexual energy towards you?

Previously, we said that true receiving is receiving everything without a point of view. "Everything" includes your sexual energy, your partner's sexual energy, and everyone else's sexual energy.

What if you could be all sexual energies and receive all sexual energies without a point of view? Receiving sexual energy does not mean you have to do anything with this energy. What if you could just enjoy the energy and allow it to contribute to you and your relationship? What if receiving anything could be as easy breathing?

Gifting Space to Your Partner

Sometimes it can be a gift to just step back and give your partner space. Two questions that you can ask are: "What will it take for me to be aware when my partner requires space?" or "Does my partner require space?"

How many of us have been taught to make it significant and wrong if our partner requires space? Remember, it's not personal or necessarily about you when your partner does require space. And when you require space you can ask for it too.

Being and Receiving Go Hand in Hand

Being and receiving go hand in hand. For instance, if you are unwilling to be kind, can you receive kindness from someone else? If you are unwilling to be vulnerable, can you receive anyone else's vulnerability?

Anything that you are unwilling to be, you cannot actually receive. Anytime you have asked for something to show up in your life and you haven't received it yet, you can ask, "What am I unwilling to be, right here and now?"

JOHN: I had been asking for a while, "What will it take to do more international workshops?" I couldn't see the possibility based on my work schedule and finances. When I first met Nirmada, I was unwilling to be vulnerable and allow myself to receive gifts from others. Once I was able to let go of this fixed point of view, I was able to receive a gift from Nirmada in the form of a flight, a workshop and the accommodations. This level of gifting and receiving created something greater for both of us.

The old paradigm is all about doing. The new paradigm is all about being all of you, asking questions and your willingness to receive. This creates the place where you open the door to new possibilities and choices beyond what you imagined was possible.

When you are following your awareness of what's light and expansive and making choices based on that, you are willing to be the energy of what you're desiring to receive. This is what allows new possibilities and choices to show up.

Summary of the Tools, Concepts and Questions from Chapter Nine

1. Questions to ask for gaining more awareness:

    - "What will it take for me to be aware of what my partner can receive?"

    - "What do I desire to receive?"

    - "What can I receive beyond what I imagined possible?"

2. Lowering your barriers for change with your partner:

    To lower your barriers, first ask for your barriers to lower and intend for them to lower. Then imagine pulling energy through the universe, through your partner and then through you. Keep doing this until your partner has also lowered their barriers and you both have a sense of peace and oneness.

3. Questions for expanding gratitude:

    • "What am I grateful for today?"

    • "What am I grateful for about me?"

    • "What am I grateful for about my partner?"

4. Questions and clearings for acknowledging your gifts:

    • "What's so easy for me to do that I don't even know it's a gift?"

    • "What are three of my gifts that I can acknowledge?"

    • "What are three of my gifts that I am grateful for?"

    • "Anything that doesn't allow me to know what my gifts are, I will now destroy and un-create it all."

5. Gifting and receiving with your sexual energy:

    • What if your sexual energy and your partner's sexual energy could be a gift to each other and to the World?

- What if your gifting and receiving of sexual energy and your partner's gifting and receiving of sexual energy were healing energies that created your new paradigm in relationship?

- And if your partner gifts their admiration to someone else, could this be a contribution to you and your relationship?

Hopefully you have been having fun playing with the tools and concepts in this chapter, and are opening yourself up to new possibilities with gifting and receiving. In the next chapter, we will be exploring more about Living in the Next 10 Seconds and Living Without Limits.

CHAPTER TEN

Living in the Next 10 Seconds

~

THIS CHAPTER IS dedicated to practicing and applying some of the key concepts we have covered throughout *Love in the Next 10 Seconds.*

This book was written for you, the reader, to know that you have choice in every 10 seconds. Have you been having fun applying the tools and questions in this book? We invite you to practice using these tools on a daily basis for creating your new paradigm of Living in the Next 10 Seconds.

Living in the Next 10 Seconds is where you let go of needing things to be either right or wrong and you are willing to make choices, 10 seconds at a time. Practicing making choices and being aware of what your choices are going to create is key in creating the future you really desire.

Choice Creates Awareness

As we continue this journey together, what new choices have you been making and what new awareness have you been receiving?

Every choice creates something, as choice is the source of creation. When you make choices beyond what you previously considered as 'right or wrong' or 'good or bad', you allow your awareness to expand for choosing what works for you, 10 seconds at a time.

With every choice you make, regardless of the outcome, you *will* gain more awareness. When you make a choice that doesn't turn out so well, a question you can ask is, "How can I use this to my advantage?" This means that you are willing to use any experience in your life to your advantage for gaining more awareness. This opens doors to new possibilities.

This is very different from taking advantage of someone, as it's about taking advantage of your own awareness. It's where you know that every challenge in your life can be used to empower you to create something beyond what you imagined was possible.

Making choices that work for you can take practice. These tools are here for you to use, so that you can know that ultimately you have unlimited choices for living without limits.

Imagine an apple tree in front of you, with each apple representing a choice. If someone told you, "You can pick any apple from the tree; however you must be blindfolded and have your hands tied behind your back," can you perceive how limiting this would be? The situation is very similar to when you cut off your awareness and stop asking questions before you make choices. Our desire is that you learn to make choices based on your awareness, 10 seconds at a time, and have access to "picking any apple that's on the tree".

When you are unclear about what your choices are creating or you require more information, you can ask, "What awareness am I having that I'm not acknowledging?" or "What information do I require?" These questions will enable you to receive more awareness and clarity.

NIRMADA: When I have an intensity or pain in my body, I will ask, "What awareness am I having that I'm not acknowledging?" Oftentimes, after asking this question, the pain will either go away or I will get an awareness of something that requires my attention.

Our bodies are sensory awareness organisms that are constantly giving us information from others and the world around us. Listening to this information and awareness, even when you have nothing to do with it, will create more ease for you and your body. Have you been listening to the information and awareness your body is giving you?

What's Right about This That I'm Not Getting?

Have you been allowing the experiences in your life to contribute to greater awareness, regardless of the outcome?

When things show up that are different than what you imagined, rather than going into wrongness and thinking that something bad has just occurred, you can ask, "What's right about this that I'm not getting?"

When you ask this question, you can use any experience in your life to gain more awareness, which then opens the door to new possibilities. When you welcome awareness, even when it is uncomfortable, it expands your reality and creates new possibilities.

If you do make yourself wrong, a quick way of changing this is to ask, "What's right about me that I'm not getting?" Asking this question can shift your perspective away from wrongness and into new possibilities. Would you be willing to ask this question so that you can remember the greatness of you?

Asking Questions for Receiving Awareness

Have you been practicing asking questions for receiving more awareness? The beauty of asking questions is that it's the key for changing anything. The more awareness you have, the better your choices will become, and the easier it will be to make choices.

It's very rare for things to show up like you imagined. However, when you are open to all possibilities and are asking questions, you allow things to be able to show up greater than you have imagined.

Remember, when you ask a question, the awareness might not come right away. For instance, you might be walking down the street two weeks after having asked a question, and you hear a child say something, and suddenly you get the awareness to the question you had asked. The receiving of awareness is not logical or cognitive, as it just comes when it comes. What question can you ask today to receive more awareness?

Making Choices in 10-Second Increments

Have you been practicing Making Choices in 10-Second Increments? When you have made choices that didn't work out so well, have you been practicing making new choices in the next 10 seconds?

When you ask questions and make choices 10 seconds at a time, you become the creator of both your own reality and your new paradigm of living without limits. Your new paradigm is about knowing you have choice, and just because you chose something in one 10 seconds, that doesn't mean that you can't choose again in the next 10 seconds. This can include choices in areas such as where you work, the relationship you are in, where you live, what you eat, and the friends you hang out with.

In this book we have talked about expanding your awareness, being willing to see things as they are, and getting out of making conclusions by asking questions. The more you practice making choices in 10-second increments, the easier it becomes to know what works for you and what doesn't work for you.

Ultimately, making choices 10 seconds at a time means that you are empowered to know that nobody else's answer is greater than your own awareness. What new choices can you make in the next 10 seconds?

Having Ease with Making Choices

Have you been practicing being at ease with making new choices?

Being at ease with making choices, in 10-second increments, comes from knowing that if you make a choice and it doesn't work out, then you can make a new choice in the next 10 seconds. In this way, you can never make a wrong choice. You get to keep choosing every 10 seconds.

The benefit of making choices, 10 seconds at a time, is that you become the creator of your own life and there is a sense of ease with the choices that you make.

Making choices with ease, 10 seconds at a time, means that you have the freedom to choose, without needing to make yourself wrong, regardless of the outcome of what your choices create.

The old paradigm teaches us to look for answers, rather than being empowered to ask questions and to trust our own knowing. It also teaches us to follow a set plan, rather than being the leader in our own lives, where we are choosing what works for us, 10 seconds at a time.

In the new paradigm, even if you have spent a long time planning something, and you suddenly realize it's not going to work, you know you have the freedom in the next 10 seconds to make a new choice. With this freedom, you become the leader in your own life by trusting your awareness, 10 seconds at time. Are you willing to be the leader in your own life?

Perceiving Your Light and Heavy

Have you been practicing with Perceiving Your Light and Heavy for making choices? This is a pragmatic tool that will guide you in making choices that work for you 10 seconds at a time.

The new paradigm is about seeing things 'as they are' and making choices based on this awareness, rather than on what you've concluded they should be. When you apply the tool of Perceiving Your Light and Heavy, it will guide you in knowing what does and doesn't work for you and allow you to make better choices.

Have you been practicing becoming aware of your body's sensations while perceiving what is light and heavy? When you listen to the information and awareness your body is giving you in this way, you can make choices from a place of expansion and possibility rather than from a place of contraction and conclusion.

The next time you are choosing something and you perceive it as heavy and contracted, would you be willing to ask a question and be aware of what your choice will create?

The next time you are choosing something and you perceive it as light and expansive, would you be willing to ask a question and be aware of what your choice will create?

What are My Choices Going to Create?

Have you been practicing being aware of what your choices are creating?

You can look at what your choices are going to create by asking:

- "If I choose this, what will my life be like in five years?"

- "If I don't choose this, what will my life be like in five years?"

These questions are a practical tool for making choices about anything in your life and relationship, without going into conclusion about what the outcome will be. These questions are not meant to conclude what your life will actually be like in five years; rather, you ask these questions so you can perceive the energy (expansive or contractive) of what your choices will create.

When you ask these two questions, you will most likely perceive one energy out of the two as lighter and more expansive, indicating what choice will work for you.

For example, if you decided to buy a house, you could ask, "If I choose to buy this house, what will my life be like in five years?" After asking this, if you perceive the energy as light and expansive, it's a clear indication that it's a choice that would work for you. Alternatively, if you were to ask, "If I don't choose to buy this house, what will my life be like in five years?" and you perceive the energy as heavy, this would be a clear indication that your choice to buy the house was going to work for you. What will it take for you to ask questions before you make important choices in your life?

Destroying and Un-creating Your Relationship Every Day

Have you been practicing destroying and un-creating your relationship every day? Every day, you can say: "Everything that my relationship was yesterday, I will now destroy and un-create it all."

Destroying and un-creating your relationship every day allows you to create your relationship anew every day *and* 10 seconds at a time. Remember, you are not *actually* destroying and un-creating the relationship. Rather, what you are destroying and un-creating are the limitations, expectations, projections, conclusions and judgments about the relationship.

What if your relationship could be new and exciting every day?

Destroying and Un-creating Limitations

Have you been practicing destroying and un-creating things that aren't working for you anymore? If you chose something in the past and it no longer works for you now, we encourage you to not go into the wrongness of the previous choices you have made. Rather, you can use this awareness to make new choices and you can always destroy and un-create any limitations that are holding the past in place.

When you destroy and un-create something that you desire to change, you are destroying and un-creating old, stuck energy that holds limitations in place, and this allows for new possibilities to arise. You can practice destroying and un-creating limitations in any area of your life that isn't working for you.

Here are some examples:

- "Everything I judged about my body, I will now destroy and un-create it all."

- "Everything I concluded about money, I will now destroy and un-create it all."

- "Everything I concluded about sex and relationship, I will now destroy and un-create it all."

What will it take for you to have fun destroying and un-creating anything that doesn't work for you?

New Awareness of Your Relational Reality

Are you now gaining more awareness of *your* relational reality?

Living in the Next 10 Seconds helps you to get clear about what *your* relational reality is. When you are creating your life 10 seconds at a time, your relational reality will move out of the box of relationship and into living without limits.

If the tools in this book are empowering you to create a great relationship, then we are happy for you. If the tools are empowering you in realizing that the relationship you are in isn't working for you, then we are equally happy for you. Either way, what we are sharing with you in this book will allow you to create your new paradigm of Living in the Next 10 Seconds.

How much fun can you have, living in the next 10 seconds?

Being Willing to Lose Anything That's Limiting You

Are you willing to lose anything that's limiting you from being all of you?

When you practice the adventure of Living in the Next 10 Seconds, you never know what's going to show up. When you are willing to let go of preconceived ideas of how things need to be, you open yourself up to a world of possibilities that you didn't even know existed.

How many of us have cut off parts and pieces of ourselves to be with another person, or to have something? The willingness to lose anyone or anything is imperative in being and in having all of you. The willingness to lose anyone or anything doesn't mean that you actually have to lose them. Whenever you are willing to lose anything, or anyone, this allows you to have greater intimacy in your life and to go deeper into asking questions for creating the future you really desire.

Are you willing to be and have all of you?

What Other Choices are Available?

Have you been asking what other choices are available for creating your life?

When things don't show up like we have imagined, it can sometimes create a situation where we become unclear about what to choose next. When you are not sure what to choose next, you can ask, "What other choices are available?" or "What other choices are available I haven't considered before?"

When you ask these questions, it changes the energy of many situations and allows you to have new choices and possibilities available to you beyond what you previously considered possible.

What new choices can you make for living without limits?

Your Point of View Creates Your Reality

Have you been making changes for creating the future you desire?

Since your point of view creates your reality, what points of view can you change that will create the future you desire? For example, if you desire a more expanded relationship, what needs to change for you to create this?

Asking questions is key for changing any situation from a limited state to an expansive space. Questions you can ask are, "What question can I ask to expand my reality?" or "What point of view can I change to expand my reality?"

Whenever you find yourself limited by a fixed point of view, you can say: "Interesting Point of View, I have this point of view," three or more times—until you notice you are becoming lighter and more expansive.

Have you been using the tool of Interesting Point of View regarding the changes in your life?

What's it Going to Take to Change This?

Have you been asking, "What's it going to take to change this?" when you desire something to change?

Asking "What will it take to change this?" or "What can I be or do today to change this right away?" are tools you can use for creating change in any area of your life. Asking these questions starts to open up the door to new possibilities for you, even if you don't get the awareness of what that is, right away.

Let's say your partner complains they don't have enough free time to get to the gym and are concerned that they never will. You can ask, "Well, what can you be or do to change this?" This question gets them contemplating other choices they could make. A while later your partner gets the awareness that they could hire an additional employee to free up their time for going to the gym.

The next time your partner complains about something, would you be willing to ask, "What's it going to take to change this?" The next time you find yourself not getting what you desire, would you be willing to ask, "What can I be or do today to change this right away?"

Acknowledgment and Gratitude

Have you been practicing acknowledging yourself and your partner and being grateful for yourself and your partner?

Acknowledgment and gratitude can be used and enjoyed on a daily basis in your life and relationship for creating something greater. Have you noticed that things have changed in your life from applying the tools of Acknowledgment and Gratitude?

Here are some questions for being grateful and practicing acknowledgment:

- "What am I grateful for about myself?"

- "What can I acknowledge about myself?"

- "What am I grateful for about my partner?"

- "What can I acknowledge about my partner?"

What Else is Possible?

Have you been expanding your life and choices by asking, "What else is possible?" We encourage you to continue being empowered to know what you know, to trust your awareness and to continue asking questions. What will it take for you to use these tools on a daily basis for changing any area of your life?

Summary of the Tools, Concepts and Questions from Chapter Ten

1. "What awareness am I having that I'm not acknowledging?" or "What information do I require?" — Questions you can ask that will enable you to receive more awareness and clarity.

2. "What's right about this that I'm not getting?" and "What's right about me that I'm not getting?" — Questions that you can ask to shift your focus from a problem, and into greater possibilities.

3. "What questions can I ask to receive more awareness?" — A question that you can ask to receive more awareness.

4. "What new choices can I make in the next 10 seconds?" — A question you can ask to keep expanding into new choices and possibilities.

5. "If I choose this, what will my life be like in five years?" and "If I don't choose this, what will my life be like in five years?" — Questions you can ask to perceive the awareness of what your choice will create.

6. Statements that allow you to destroy and un-create limitations in any area of your life:

   - "Everything I judged about my body, I will now destroy and un-create it all."

   - "Everything I concluded about money, I will now destroy and un-create it all."

   - "Everything I concluded about sex and relationship, I will now destroy and un-create it all."

7. "What other choices are available?" or "What other choices are available that I haven't considered before?" — Questions you can ask for expanding your choices.

8. "Interesting Point of View, I have this point of view." — A phrase that you can say to dissipate any limiting point of view.

9. "What's it going to take to change this?" — A question you can ask of any situation that isn't working that you would like to change.

10. Questions that you can ask to create something greater for yourself and with your partner:

    •   "What am I grateful for about myself?"

    •   "What can I acknowledge about myself?"

    •   "What am I grateful for about my partner?"

    •   "What can I acknowledge about my partner?"

Now that we have reviewed some of the key tools in this book, in the next chapter we will explore using the tool of Acknowledgment on a deeper level, and the tool of Admiration, which creates more intimacy with your partner.

CHAPTER ELEVEN

Practicing Acknowledgment and Admiration

~

IN YOUR NEW paradigm, acknowledgment and admiration are tools you can use daily and 10 seconds at a time. Acknowledgment can be a way of showing your appreciation and gratitude for yourself and your partner. Admiration allows you to have the pleasure and appreciation of receiving anyone or anything without barriers.

Acknowledgment and admiration can be used with your partner when things are going well and when things are challenging. The opposite of acknowledgment is rejection and the opposite of admiration is criticism. Using these tools is a way of eliminating separation from your partner as well as getting out of the box of relationship and into living without limits.

When you practice acknowledging what is going well, it allows for more of the good things to show up. When you practice admiration, you lower your barriers and expand your receiving.

Acknowledging and Admiring Yourself

Acknowledging and admiring yourself is one of the greatest ways to increase being all of you. Did anyone ever teach you to acknowledge or admire yourself as a child? What if you could now practice acknowledging and admiring yourself daily, and by doing so you could rediscover capabilities you didn't realize you had?

When you acknowledge yourself, you are honoring what is true for you. Admiring yourself allows you to have easy access to who you can become in each 10 seconds.

AN EXERCISE IN ACKNOWLEDGING AND ADMIRING YOURSELF

If you find it easy to acknowledge children, practice acknowledging yourself with the same tenderness as you do towards them.

- What are three things you can acknowledge about yourself?

- What are three things you can acknowledge about your body?

- What are three things you admire about yourself?

- What are three things you admire about your body?

Notice what changes and expands as you acknowledge and admire yourself.

Acknowledging and Admiring Your Partner

Acknowledging and admiring your partner means you are aware of where they are at in every 10 seconds and that you have allowance for what they are choosing. You can continue to encourage them to expand into something greater, while having no barriers up to them and what they are choosing.

JOHN: When I met Nirmada, she began acknowledging many things about me. She would acknowledge, for example, my kindness, healing capacities with bodies and that I was a great dad. At first, this was new to me in a relationship. However, I would receive what she had acknowledged and began to notice how it created more awareness and expansion in those areas. One of the things that I am so grateful to Nirmada for is all the acknowledgment she has given to me in many areas of my life.

NIRMADA: John has so many talents and capacities that I can see in him, and by acknowledging and admiring them, something greater is created for both of us.

AN EXERCISE IN ADMIRING YOUR PARTNER

- What are three things you admire about your partner?

- What are three things you admire about your partner's body?

- What are three things you admire about your relationship?

Acknowledgment and Inspiration

In our relationship, we have used acknowledging each other as a way of inspiring ourselves to recognize our gifts and to enable each of us to continue to choose to create the future we really desire. What can you acknowledge about your partner that will inspire you to choose more for you?

NIRMADA: John and I are both into holistic living and taking good care of our bodies. We often acknowledge each other for this and it inspires both of us to take better care of ourselves and our bodies.

JOHN: When I first met Nirmada, I was delighted to discover that she had received so much bodywork, including gifting and receiving of Bars. This has inspired me and many other people to choose to receive more bodywork too.

Acknowledgment and Family

Oprah Winfrey had a guest on her show who talked about having a book in which he and his family wrote acknowledgments. The book showed how everyone in the family practiced acknowledging each other, rather than judging each other. This changed the ways in which his whole family related and contributed to one another.

Imagine if every family had a book of acknowledgments like this. What if you could practice acknowledging everyone in your life?

Admiration for Undoing Conflict

You can use admiration in the midst of a conflict for changing the energy. When you do so, it is a way of bringing more expansion to the moment, and closing the perceived gap of separation between you and your partner.

The next time you and your partner are having a conflict, you can pause, and practice admiring three things about each other and allow your barriers to lower.

NIRMADA AND JOHN: We knew a couple that had just had a baby. The mother was frantic trying to take care of the baby, breastfeeding, keeping the house clean, and making sure the other children were also taken care of. One night, her husband came home from work and the stress level was so high that the two of them began to argue.

He finally realized that the level of pressure his wife was under was unbearable for her, so he stopped arguing. Instead, he began admiring her for being an incredible wife and an amazing caretaker of their children. As she received this admiration, she melted into his arms and the conflict was completely gone.

Acknowledgment and Allowance for 'What Is'

One of the keys for creating what you desire is acknowledging and having allowance for 'what is', rather than having a point of view about what you think things should be. You may see things that are not always comfortable and you may also be pleasantly surprised by what you see.

Asking questions, acknowledging what you know, and being in the question of "What else is possible?" is how you create freedom and choice for yourself, regardless of what other people choose. When you acknowledge what you are aware of, it gets you present with where you are now and with the new choices you can make.

Gary used this tool to see his relationship with his second wife more clearly. After several years of being with her, he realized that there were eight things that would need to change in order for the relationship to work for him. He became aware that if he asked her to change six of these, it would be like asking a leopard to change its spots. He finally acknowledged that she was not capable of changing these things and that the relationship wasn't going to work anymore.

If you have been cutting off your awareness about what actually works for you, a question you can ask is "What awareness do I have that I'm not acknowledging?" Asking this question will allow you to receive more awareness and gain more clarity.

Acknowledging What's Vital to You

When something is vital to you, it means that it's essential for your well-being and that it is something you would desire not to live without. Acknowledging what's vital to you will contribute to gaining more awareness and making choices that work for you. You can also ask your partner what's vital to them, so you both gain more awareness and clarity.

NIRMADA: What's vital to me is creating more consciousness everywhere I can, while having fun doing so, and having a partner that shares these values.

JOHN: What's vital to me is that my partner has to be nurturing of my body, is able to receive me and that I'm able to receive them.

The Power of Positive Acknowledgment

Dr. Masaru Emoto carried out another experiment on positive and negative energies. He placed portions of cooked rice into two jars. On one jar he wrote 'thank you', and on the other jar he wrote 'you fool'. He then instructed school children to say out loud every day what was written on the labels of the jars, as they passed by them. After 30 days, the rice in the jar with the positive acknowledgment of 'thank you' had barely changed, while the rice in the other jar was moldy and rotten.

Practicing Acknowledgment and Admiration

How much fun can you have practicing acknowledgment and admiration every day? What if every day you could acknowledge and admire: your body, your partner's body, having used the tools in this book, things you have already changed, that you are choosing a more conscious relationship, the gift you are to the world, and so on...

We would also like to acknowledge and admire you for using the tools in this book for creating more consciousness and awareness for yourself and the contribution that is to the World.

Summary of the Tools, Concepts and Questions from Chapter Eleven

1. When you acknowledge yourself, you are honoring what is true for you. Admiring yourself allows you to have easy access to who you can become in each 10 seconds.

2. Questions for acknowledging and admiring yourself:

    •   "What are three things I can acknowledge about myself?"

    •   "What are three things I admire about myself?"

3. Acknowledging and admiring your partner is also being aware of where they are at in each 10 seconds, and having allowance for what they are choosing.

4. Questions for admiring your partner:

   • "What are three things I admire about my partner?"

   • "What are three things I admire about my partner's body?"

5. The next time you and your partner are having a conflict, you can pause, and practice admiring three things about each other and allow your barriers to lower.

6. "What awareness do I have that I'm not acknowledging?" — Asking this question will allow you to receive more awareness and gain more clarity.

7. Acknowledging what's vital to you will contribute to gaining more awareness and to making choices that work for you.

8. "How much fun can I have practicing acknowledgment and admiration every day?" — A question you can ask yourself daily.

Hopefully you have been practicing acknowledgment and admiration on a daily basis and opening yourself up to new possibilities. We are going to continue to guide you in the adventure of living without limits as we move into the final chapter, where we will be exploring what you and your partner can create together.

CHAPTER TWELVE

What Can We Create Together?

~

IN THIS FINAL chapter, we are going to explore how to create your relationship as a working possibility. When you want to know if your relationship is a working possibility, you look at what's actually possible with your partner. This is also where you *actually* see your partner *as* they are, rather than expecting them to be somebody that they're not.

The new paradigm is about letting go of requiring your partner to do the things you want them to do and always making it about giving them choice. When a relationship is a working possibility, you are creating a relationship, rather than 'having' a relationship.

Changing the Box of Relationship

"Changing the Box of Relationship" is where you get out of putting limitations on what your relationship is supposed to be. It is also about creating beyond what you and your partner have allowed yourselves to be or do within the relationship.

It means no longer needing to cut off parts and pieces of yourself in order to be in the relationship, and not expecting your partner to do so either. It also means that you and your partner have the choice to be yourselves, 10 seconds at a time.

Living Without Limits

"Living Without Limits" in your new paradigm is like being a kid in a candy store. How much fun can you have on the adventure of creating your life and living without limits? If you really desire to create your life, it's essential to function from question, choice, possibility, and contribution.

Asking questions is for gaining more awareness and opening doors to new possibilities. Choice creates awareness. If you are truly willing to function from question, choice, and possibility, then you begin to open doors to things you never before considered were possible. When you allow everything in your life to contribute to you, new possibilities will arrive for living without limits.

What Can We Create Together?

The new paradigm allows you to expand your creative capacities in your relationship, and, unlike the old paradigm, to create beyond making babies and renovating houses.

In many relationships, when people first get together, they often have what is known as the 'honeymoon period'. At the beginning, couples often find that they are in the magic of creation mode. There is a sense that anything is possible as their two energies come together and intertwine.

This magic of creating together can often wear off when the partners start to maintain the status quo, having stopped asking questions and having put the relationship into a box. What if instead they could continue the adventure of the magic and creating together?

It's similar to when you move to a new town or city — in the first few weeks, you find yourself totally open to all the possibilities your new environment is offering. You make new friends, for example, you go to new classes, and explore different areas.

You are probably alive and present to all that is being offered. Then gradually, as time goes on, you start to get into a routine and stop exploring. Maybe months later, or even years later, you discover something that was right around your corner that you didn't even know existed. You were so caught up in your routine or pattern that your awareness was closed off to experiencing new possibilities.

Relationship in the old paradigm can be very similar to this. When we first connect with someone, we are open to all the possibilities that the relationship has to offer and are excited to explore new things. Eventually, many people retreat into their familiar patterns and as a result may start maintaining the relationship rather than creating it.

By applying the tools in this book, you can continue to explore new possibilities in creating your relationship 10 seconds at time.

NIRMADA: A client of mine was interested in a woman who wanted him to commit to having a child within the first year of the marriage. He just wanted to enjoy her. However, she was attached to her conclusion about what she needed to create in the relationship. This became a huge source of contention between them. He agreed to revisit their discussion of having a child after they were married for one year. In the meantime, they ended up renovating a house.

Both of them were committed. However, their commitment was to the conclusion that they should stay together, which is why they ended up marrying each other, despite having challenges. Neither of them was able to change the box of relationship and see what else they could create together.

They were divorced within a year of getting married. However, they both had divorced themselves by cutting off parts and pieces of themselves, long before the relationship ended.

Can you imagine how different their choices would have been if they had asked a question like "If I choose to marry this person what will my life be like in five years?" before they entered into the marriage?

What Would Be Fun for Us to Create Together?

A question you can ask every day is "What would be fun for us to create together today?" When you ask this question, you will start to receive new awareness of different choices and possibilities you have with your partner. So, what will it take for you to have more fun than you imagined creating with your partner?

NIRMADA: When John and I first met, we realized right away that we had the capacity to create together. We started asking, "What would be fun for us to create together?" By asking this question, *Love in the Next 10 Seconds*, among many other things, was created.

Being the Creator of Your Own Reality

When we speak about creation, it is worth noting that everyone is creating all of the time. Every choice you make creates something. As we previously highlighted, "Your point of view creates your reality."

The question is "What are you creating with the choices you are making?" Are you creating something greater from the choices you are making, or are you creating undesirable moments in your life from the choices you are making?

As previously highlighted, you can ask, "If I choose this, what will my life be like in five years?" Asking this question allows you to perceive the energy of what your choices will create and what's light and expansive for you to choose.

Being the Leader in Your Own Life

Being the leader in your own life means that you are going where you are going, regardless of whether anyone else comes or not. It's where you are choosing what you are choosing, regardless of what other people choose.

Making choices is not *always* easy. However, when you are the leader in your own life, and are following the energy of what's light and expansive, you will be able to continue making choices 10 seconds at a time.

Are you willing to be the leader in your own life?

Creating a World You Would Like to Live In

Creating in the new paradigm is about continuously asking, "What can we create together?" It's about creating new possibilities and creating beyond your current reality.

It's also about what you can create in communion with the Earth. Living your new paradigm of relationship is a huge contribution to the Earth! If everybody on the planet functioned from outside the box of relationship, this would likely create more of the kind of World that we would all desire to live in.

NIRMADA: John and I share similar values — to create more consciousness everywhere we can, and to have fun doing so. We do this individually and together, and it contributes to creating a World we desire to live in.

JOHN: Being with Nirmada is a reality changing choice, which includes the Earth and everyone on it. For us, there are no limitations as to what we can create together.

Living Beyond Definition

"Definition, by definition alone, is limitation." Gary Douglas

Imagine what your relationship would be like if you didn't have to define it and put it in a box? Imagine what your life would be like if you no longer had to define yourself?

Living beyond definition means that you don't conclude what will show up and you are always in the question of "What else is possible?" Living beyond definition also means you are open to the possibility that things might not show up as you imagined.

When you live beyond definition, you may even choose to not define your relationship *as* a relationship. What if, instead, you were just making the choice to be together, 10 seconds at a time? Can you perceive how much more space this would make for creating together?

NIRMADA: We have interviewed many couples that are creating their new paradigm of relationship. When we asked one couple how they would characterize their relationship, they said, "We wouldn't. It's indefinable. It's just a choice that we are together, even though we have been making that choice for 45 years. It is such a freedom to know that we always have choice." They described how they are not locked into the relationship with expectations and projections, and are instead making the choice to be together 10 seconds at a time.

Choosing Relationships that Contribute to Your Life

A great question to ask about every person in your life is "Does having this person in my life actually expand my life and contribute to me?" What if every person in your life could add to your life and contribute to you? If someone is not adding to your life or contributing to you, you may want to ask yourself, "What other choices are available?"

NIRMADA: Shortly after I started expanding my awareness and changing at a fast rate, many of my close friends stopped wanting to hang out with me. After I got over the initial surprise, I began to realize that they didn't desire to change and grow in the same way that I did, and do.

Ultimately, this was a gift, as it freed up my energy to create my life in new ways. I became aware that no longer having these people in my daily life made it easier, as they weren't adding to, or contributing to, what I was choosing.

Creating from Choice 10 Seconds at a Time

Every choice you make creates something new. Every 10 seconds you have the choice to create your relationship and also to create something greater. Remember, a choice is only good for 10 seconds. It's now a new 10 seconds and you can choose again. If you choose to create your life and your relationship 10 seconds at a time, you get to keep choosing new possibilities.

If you had 10 seconds to live the rest of your life, what would you choose? Now that 10 seconds is up, what else would you choose? Would you consider allowing life to unfold in this way and ride the wave of possibility with creating your life 10 seconds at a time? What if the purpose of life is to have fun? What can you choose today so that you can have more fun right away??

What Would I Really Like to Create?

If you had $100,000,000 put into your bank account at the beginning of every year for the rest of your life, what would you choose to create?

Questions for gaining more awareness:

- "If money weren't the issue, what would I choose to create?"

- "If time weren't the issue, what would I choose to create?"

- "If family weren't the issue, what would I choose to create?"

Creation and The Kingdom of We

Some couples really enjoy working and creating together, and others know it just doesn't work for them. What if there were no right or wrong, and it was just a choice? You may realize that you do not desire to do everything with your partner.

When you choose to do things individually, you can still support each other energetically. As we highlighted previously, this is known as The Kingdom of We, rather than The Kingdom of Me.

When you choose to create from The Kingdom of We, you are including your partner in your choices. This is where you allow them to energetically contribute to you and you can also energetically contribute to them.

When your creations are going well and you desire more to show up, you can ask:

- "What else is possible?"

- "How does it get any better than this?"

When your creations aren't going so well and you desire something better to show up, you can ask:

- "What's it going to take to change this?"

- "What else is possible?"

- "How does it get any better than this?"

All of Life Comes to Me with Ease, Joy and Glory®

In the closing of this book, we wish to present you with one more special tool, which is to repeat the following phrase, silently or out loud, 10 times in the morning and 10 times in the evening: "All of life comes to me with ease, joy and glory."

This is a tool from Access Consciousness, and by saying it often, it can truly create more ease, more joy and more glory in every area of your life and relationship. This doesn't mean that things will always be easy.

What it does mean is that you will have more ease with whatever shows up.

Now that you have read *Love in the Next 10 Seconds* and received some amazing tools, our question to you is, "If you could create anything in your life and relationship, what would it be?"

Summary of the Tools, Concepts and Questions from Chapter Twelve

1. Creating a working possibility in relationship — Where you look at what's actually possible with your partner and where you *actually* see your partner *as* they are, rather than expecting them to be somebody that they're not.

2. "What can we create together?" — A question you can ask daily for gaining more awareness about what you can create with your partner.

3. "What would be fun for us to create together today?" — A question you can ask that will allow you to receive new awareness of different choices and possibilities you have with your partner.

4. "What am I creating with the choices I am making?" — A question you can ask to become more aware of what your choices are creating.

5. Being the leader in your own life — A phrase that means that you are going where you are going, regardless of whether anyone else comes or not.

6. Imagine what your relationship would be like if you didn't have to define it and put it in a box?

7. "Does having this person in my life actually expand my life and contribute to me?" — A question to ask to ensure that you are choosing relationships that are expansive and that contribute to you.

8. "All of life comes to me with ease, joy and glory." — A special phrase which you can repeat, silently or out loud, 10 times in the morning and 10 times in the evening. By saying this often it can truly create more ease, more joy and more glory in every area of your life and relationship.

It is our wish that this final chapter has given you tools to expand what you can create for yourself and what you can create in your new paradigm of relationship.

In the next section of the book, to further contribute to your living without limits, we will share with you "What's Next and What Else is Possible?" and the continuation of our journey together...

WHAT'S NEXT AND WHAT ELSE IS POSSIBLE?

~

CONGRATULATIONS! YOU HAVE now read *Love in the Next 10 Seconds* and your journey continues for living without limits! We encourage you to play with, practice and have fun using these tools on a daily basis. You can use this book as a reference guide for your ongoing journey of loving and living in the next 10 seconds.

For us, using these tools has been an ongoing journey of loving and living 10 seconds at a time. We have learned that a choice is truly only good for 10 seconds. So, when we make choices that don't *always* work for us, we know that we can make a new choice again in the next 10 seconds.

This book is our gift to the World for creating a more harmonious planet, one relationship at a time. We desire for you to know that in every 10 seconds you have the choice to be all of you, whether you are in relationship or not.

What if you could create your relationship 10 seconds at a time, without cutting off any parts of yourself? Having allowance for who your partner is, and for what they choose, will ultimately create freedom and ease for you.

When your relationship is a working possibility, it adds to your life rather than becoming your life. It's where you are contributing to each other on a daily basis and this creates a dynamic working possibility. What if you could do 'relationship light' instead of 'relationship right'?

Our Journey Continues...

One year after we first met, we returned to our meeting place in Costa Rica for a special event called *The Living Dream*. The joy of our reunion was a testimony to how much we had both changed and how using the tools contained in this book had contributed to our journey of living without limits.

We are creating our relationship as a working possibility and it is indefinable. Making choices in 10-second increments has allowed us to continuously create a relationship that works for us. We have learned to not make conclusions about what our relationship should be, and this allows us to change, grow and thrive 10 seconds at a time.

As we continue to create the future we really desire, we don't have a preconceived idea of what shape our relationship will take. We are present with each other moment to moment and making choices that work for us by loving and living 10 seconds at time.

May all of life come to you with ease, joy and glory.

With infinite gratitude,

Nirmada & John

RESOURCES

~

1. If you would like to contact Nirmada Kaufman
   for private sessions or Access Consciousness
   Workshops, please visit: www.RadicalDemand.com
   or www.nirmadakaufman.accessconsciousness.com

2. If you would like to contact John Andros for
   private sessions or Access Consciousness
   Workshops, please visit: www.JohnAndros.net or
   www.johnandros.accessconsciousness.com

3. To learn more or join the *Love in the Next 10 Seconds*
   Book Club, please visit:
   LoveInTheNext10Seconds.com/BookClub

4. If you enjoyed reading this book and would like
   to know more about Access Consciousness®,
   please visit: http://accessconsciousness.com

5. Access Bars® is easy to learn and a fun and
   delightful activity that you can enjoy and share
   with your partner or anyone else. If you are

interested in learning more, please visit: http://bars.accessconsciousness.com

Here's a link to locate a Certified Bars Practitioner in your area: http://www.bars. accessconsciousness.com/facilitators.asp

6. If you are interested in knowing more about The Access Consciousness Clearing Statement, please visit: http://www.theclearingstatement.com

7. Let us know your feedback! Join the conversation here:

Facebook: Love in the Next 10 Seconds

Twitter: @LoveIn10Seconds

YouTube Channel: Love in the Next 10 Seconds

ABOUT THE AUTHORS

~

NIRMADA KAUFMAN and JOHN ANDROS, authors of *Love in the Next 10 Seconds*, are catalysts for consciousness. They work with clients around the world, guiding them to create radically different relationships and lives.

Their book was inspired by the question, *"What contribution can we be to ease the pain between men and women on this planet?"* Their book and businesses are their own personal contributions to creating greater harmony on the planet, one relationship at a time.

At the very beginning of their relationship, Nirmada and John discovered they had a shared love of learning, growing and consciousness. With a personal desire to create greater health and wellness in their own lives and in the lives of others, they sought out, and trained in, many different healing modalities. They bring together all these different modalities in their work with clients both through hands-on healing and in virtual sessions worldwide.

As partners in consciousness, Nirmada and John choose to create their relationship 10 seconds at a time. They refer daily to the tools in their own book. Every day they make the choice to embody these tools and the ease and communion that are possible when using them.

~

NIRMADA KAUFMAN, The Radical Demand Diva, is a #1 Bestselling Author, Pragmatic Futurist and an Access Consciousness® Certified Facilitator. She is best known for empowering and facilitating the seekers around the world who are demanding change and are ready for it now. Using a radically effective and pragmatic approach, she guides her clients to be a Radical Demand for themselves so that they can create the life and future they really desire. Through her hands-on energy work and dynamic facilitation (both virtually and in person) she's touched the lives of thousands of people around the world.

JOHN ANDROS is an author, Access Consciousness® Certified Facilitator, coach and hands-on healing practitioner. He guides clients in unwinding the stress from their bodies. He has a specialty for tapping his clients into greater choice and possibility, which leads to more ease and harmony. He empowers his clients to return home to themselves and to living without limits.

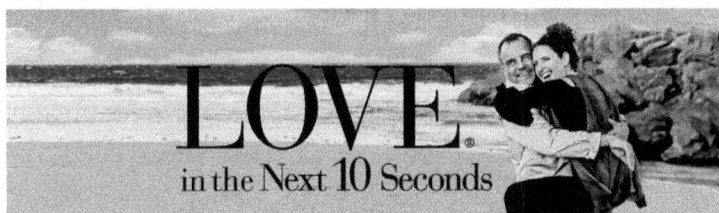

LOVE IN THE NEXT 10 SECONDS
BOOK CLUB!

~

You are invited to be a member of our *Love in the Next 10 Seconds* **Book Club** when you own a copy of our book, *Love in the Next 10 Seconds.*

We know you will receive a great deal of value from reading our book on your own and applying the dynamic tools we share to your own life.

We also know more is possible for you when you receive facilitation directly from us, the authors!

We created this **Book Club** for you, to invite you to go deeper into the topics in our book in a nurturing group environment.

When you join the *Love in the Next 10 Seconds* **Book Club**, you'll be able to join us for a *Love in the Next 10*

Seconds **Free Monthly Group Call,** on the last Tuesday of every month at 5 p.m. PST.

In this one-hour call, the lines will be open so you can ask questions, receive facilitation and explore the book topics on a deeper and more personal level. This FREE call is a great way to receive additional support and inspiration for living without limits.

BONUS: All of our calls will be recorded so, if you miss a call or wish to listen to a call again, you will have easy access to our library of archived recordings.

The *Love in the Next 10 Seconds* Book Club is for all those seeking radical change. You will learn in greater detail how to apply the tools that we share in our book in your daily life.

This is our gift for guiding you in receiving as much as possible from *Love in the Next 10 Seconds: Changing the Box of Relationship Into Living Without Limits.*

To become a member of the *Love in the Next 10 Seconds* **Book Club,** sign up here:

LoveInTheNext10Seconds.com/BookClub

When you put this book into action you will get results!

www.ingramcontent.com/pod-product-compliance
Lightning Source LLC
Chambersburg PA
CBHW060005100426
42740CB00010B/1398